MANAGEMENT OF DIABETES IN ADULTS

H. Peter Chase, MD

Satish K. Garg, MD

Library of Congress Control Number 2013939559

ISBN 9780983265030

Published by
Children's Diabetes Foundation
4380 South Syracuse Street, Suite 430
Denver, CO 80237
303-863-1200
www.ChildrensDiabetesFoundation.org

Book Design by Cynthia Kalkofen

Printed in the United States of America
by American Web

Front Cover Photos
Top left: © Rob Bum/Shutterstock
Top center: © Serp/Shutterstock
Top right: © Bochkarev Photography/Shutterstock
Bottom: © Izf/Shutterstock

Back Cover Photo © Martin Crabb

DEDICATION

This book is dedicated to our friend and colleague,
George Eisenbarth MD, Ph.D (1947-2012).

His compassionate leadership over the past 20 years
inspired the Barbara Davis Center for Diabetes
to flourish and to be a pioneer
in world-class clinical care and research.

H. Peter Chase, MD

Satish K. Garg, MD

TABLE OF CONTENTS

APPRECIATION IS EXPRESSED FOR EDITING, PROOFREADING AND MANUSCRIPT PREPARATION

Linda Chase, RN, Erin C. Cobry, MD,
Dena Gottesman, MS, RD, CDE, Cynthia Kalkofon,
Laurel Messer, RN, MPH, CDE, Sue Palandri,
Jaime Realsen, BS, Rick Realsen, R. Ph., Regina Reece,
Philip Walravens, MD and Emily Westfall, BS, BA

A special appreciation to Patricia Chase Hamilton, BA
and Jana Zinser for editing the entire publication.

OUR PURPOSE

The purpose of this book is to provide education in a simplified form for adults with type 1 or type 2 diabetes. Included are the essentials for understanding and treating adult diabetes.

When we refer to our "Center," we are referring to The Barbara Davis Center for Diabetes (www.barbaradaviscenter.org), located in Colorado. The Center follows more than 6,000 patients of all ages with both types of diabetes. We occasionally refer to methods used at our Center. However, physicians at other clinics may have different opinions regarding care and treatment. You should always follow the advice of your own diabetes care-providers.

THE IMPORTANCE OF EDUCATION

CHAPTER 1

INTRODUCTION

Diabetes terminology can be confusing. Type 2 diabetes, also known as "adult-onset diabetes," is the most common type of diabetes found world-wide. Although it is called "adult-onset," it can occur in youth (especially overweight teenagers). It is also referred to as "non-insulin dependent diabetes mellitus." However, 25 percent of people currently receive insulin. "Type 2 diabetes" is now the preferred term.

Type 1 diabetes, also known as "juvenile" or "childhood" diabetes, is the most common type of diabetes diagnosed in children and adolescents. However, it can also occur in adults. Because the adult years make up most of our lifespan, there are more people with type 1 diabetes who are adults compared to those who are below 18 years old. "Type 1 diabetes" is now the preferred term.

INITIAL EDUCATION

There was a day when people diagnosed with type 2 diabetes were told they had diabetes, given medicine and sent home without any formal education. Patients who were not given thorough education often did not do well. Education is as important for people with type 2 diabetes (and pre-type 2 diabetes) as it is for those with type 1 diabetes.

A familiar Chinese proverb says:
Give a man a fish and you feed him for a day.
Teach a man to fish and you feed him for a lifetime.

Similarly, a diabetes proverb might be:
Give a pill or a shot of insulin and sugar levels may be controlled for a day.
Give diabetes education and sugar levels may be controlled for a lifetime.

1

Diabetes education helps the person and their family to have the knowledge and skills needed to perform self-care, manage problems, and most importantly, to make lifestyle changes needed to effectively manage their diabetes.

It is now known that better sugar (glucose)* control will help prevent the complications of diabetes later in life (Chapters 16 and 17). It is also known that some people with pre-diabetes can prevent and/or delay its onset following the same treatment for people who already have type 2 diabetes (Chapters 2, 5 and 18). However, this is not likely to occur without education.

Education for type 2 diabetes (and type 1 diabetes) can be done on a one-on-one basis or in a group setting. A group setting allows support from others who have the same condition. It is also more efficient for the diabetes educators. However, one-on-one education can focus on individual problems. Healthcare-providers doing the education may include a nurse, dietitian, physician, pharmacist, psych/social person and/or exercise specialist. Follow-up appointments are best if they include one-on-one time with the healthcare-provider.

TOPICS FOR EDUCATION

Use of this book should supplement but not replace in-clinic education. Some of the topics covered in this book and in initial and follow-up appointments are outlined below:

❑ What Is Diabetes and What Causes It

❑ Food Selection
   • Types
   • Portion size
   • Weight-loss goal (if needed)

❑ The Importance of Exercise
   • Frequency
   • Duration
   • Types of appropriate exercise

❑ Oral Medications (if used)
   • Dose
   • Actions
   • Side effects
   • Effects on other medicines

*There are many types of sugars. The sugar that is elevated in diabetes is called 'glucose.' For purposes of this book we will use 'sugar' or 'glucose' to mean the same.

- ❑ Insulin (if used)
  - Method to administer (and when)
  - Types and action
  - Dose
- ❑ Blood Sugar Checking
  - Device use/types
  - Frequency
  - Desired range

- ❑ Low Blood Sugar (Hypoglycemia)
  - Signs and symptoms
  - Treatment

- ❑ High Blood Sugar (Hyperglycemia)
  - Signs and symptoms
  - Treatment

- ❑ Ketones, Diabetic Ketoacidosis (DKA) and Hyperosmolar Hyperglycemic State (HHS)
  - When to check?
  - How to handle?

- ❑ Long Term Management Goals
  - HbA1c levels (including desired range)
  - Blood pressure
  - Blood lipids (cholesterol)
  - Weight
  - Clinic visit frequency

- ❑ Sick-day and Surgery Management

- ❑ Psych/social Adjustment

- ❑ Diabetes Complications

- ❑ Diabetes Research

CONTINUING EDUCATION

Following initial education, it is essential the patient and family have regularly scheduled clinic visits. If this does not happen, the likelihood of success is very low. The frequency will vary for different patients and families, but is often every month initially. Visits may then gradually extend to every three months and sometimes to every six months.

A family that is supportive and willing to learn is very helpful for optimal diabetes care. Diabetes is a unique disease in that most of the management is done in the home-setting. Family members (with the patient's permission) can help with many areas of care. These may include making appropriate food purchases, medication reminders, helping to maintain supplies, attending clinic visits and understanding prevention of acute complications such as low blood sugar (especially if on insulin) or high blood sugar or ketone levels. When possible, a friend or family member exercising regularly with the person with diabetes may be a key to successful weight management/loss.

PSYCH/SOCIAL CONSIDERATIONS

The diagnosis of any serious disease, including diabetes, is stressful for the affected person as well as for the entire family. The initial stress may make it more difficult to learn all that is needed to manage diabetes. This gets better over time as everyone accepts and becomes more comfortable with the diagnosis. Some of the psych/social aspects of diabetes are discussed in Chapter 14. Meeting with a person trained in the psych/social aspects of diabetes can greatly aid with acceptance.

SUMMARY

Initial and continuing education are essential for people diagnosed with diabetes and pre-diabetes. Support from family members and friends is helpful in promoting good diabetes care.

WHAT IS TYPE 2 DIABETES? *Causes, Symptoms, and Diagnosis*

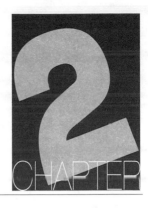

CHAPTER 2

RISK FACTORS

Risk factors for type 2 diabetes include:

- obesity (high Body Mass Index [BMI]; see Figure 1)
- high abdominal fat (waist measurement at navel more than 40 inches [100 cm])
- lack of exercise (less than 90 minutes per week)
- poor diet (high calorie, high fat)
- age (over 45 years)
- genetics (family member with type 2 diabetes)
- previous gestational diabetes (diabetes diagnosed in pregnancy)

Although obesity is a strong risk factor, not everyone with obesity has type 2 diabetes. Likewise, not everyone with type 2 diabetes is obese.

Diabetes is a condition in which the body cannot use sugar for energy. Insulin is a hormone that allows sugar to pass from the blood into body cells to be used for energy. In type 2 diabetes, there are several changes that interfere with this process.

- **Insulin Resistance:** This means the body does not respond as effectively as it should to insulin. As a result, the body cells do not get the sugar they need for energy. When this occurs, the body must produce more and more insulin to maintain a normal blood sugar level. This results in progressively higher insulin levels.

- **Glucagon:** There is an abnormal rise in glucagon levels after meals. Glucagon is a hormone that causes the liver to release more sugar into the bloodstream. Normally, glucagon levels go down after meals.

- **Decreasing Insulin Production:** Eventually, the body (pancreas) is not able to make enough insulin to maintain normal blood sugar levels. This may result in the need for insulin injections, as in patients with type 1 diabetes.

5

FIGURE 1

Body Mass Index (BMI)

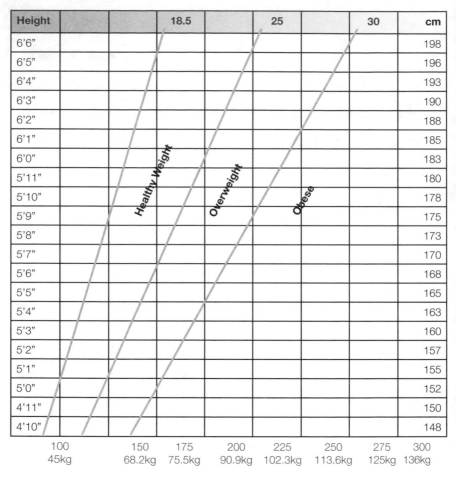

Height			18.5		25		30	cm
6'6"								198
6'5"								196
6'4"								193
6'3"								190
6'2"								188
6'1"								185
6'0"								183
5'11"								180
5'10"								178
5'9"								175
5'8"								173
5'7"								170
5'6"								168
5'5"								165
5'4"								163
5'3"								160
5'2"								157
5'1"								155
5'0"								152
4'11"								150
4'10"								148

| 100 | | 150 | 175 | 200 | 225 | 250 | 275 | 300 |
| 45kg | | 68.2kg | 75.5kg | 90.9kg | 102.3kg | 113.6kg | 125kg | 136kg |

Pounds
(Kg)

The BMI relates weight to height. To determine your BMI, find your height to the left (inches) or right (centimeters) and track horizontally to where your weight (below) intersects. Your BMI range is then shown at the top.

6

SYMPTOMS

Symptoms may initially be noticed during a period of stress or illness. However, since the onset of type 2 diabetes is often very slow, many people don't notice any symptoms before they are diagnosed. Many people with type 2 diabetes are diagnosed because a high blood sugar level was found during routine check-ups.

The symptoms of diabetes are caused by elevated blood sugar levels and thus are the same for both types of diabetes. Some of the most common symptoms of diabetes are:

- frequent urination (polyuria)

- frequent drinking of liquids (polydipsia)

- eating more and still feeling hungry (polyphagia)

- weight loss (especially in type 1 diabetes) at the time of diagnosis

- less energy

- headaches

- blurred vision

- tingling or strange feelings in toes/feet

The reason why diabetes causes frequent urination is that the kidneys pass the excess sugar from the bloodstream into the urine. Water must go out with the sugar, so urination is increased. Frequent drinking of fluids then occurs to replace the water lost as a result of the frequent urination. Weight gain (initially) is from excess eating as the body cannot use sugar for energy (due to a lack of insulin activity) and gives a message to eat more. At a later stage, body fat and protein are broken down for energy, resulting in weight loss (although weight loss is more common for people with type 1 diabetes).

PRE-TYPE 2 DIABETES

It is important to remember that many people with type 2 diabetes have a slow onset of diabetes and they may not have any symptoms. This is particularly true with a condition called "pre-diabetes." It may be harder to take the diagnosis seriously when there are no symptoms to be reversed by treatment.

People with pre-diabetes outnumber those who have type 2 diabetes. The diagnosis is based on 'borderline' blood sugar levels (Table 1).

The blood sugar levels are above normal, but are not high enough to diagnose diabetes. It is important to know who has pre-diabetes, as treatment may help them to delay or prevent the onset of type 2 diabetes. Similar methods (blood sugar [glucose] levels and HbA1c values) are used for the diagnosis of pre-diabetes or of diabetes. Pre-type 2 diabetes is discussed in more detail in Chapter 18, Type 2 Diabetes Research.

Metabolic Syndrome

Some people with pre-diabetes also have what is called "metabolic syndrome." Metabolic syndrome is a combination of problems including high abdominal fat (increased waist circumference at the navel provides a rough estimate), insulin resistance, high blood pressure, increased triglyceride and decreased High-Density Lipoprotein (HDL). Metabolic syndrome is considered a risk factor for both type 2 diabetes and for cardiovascular disease.

DIAGNOSIS AND LABORATORY VALUES

Conditions used to diagnose diabetes, as recommended by the American Diabetes Association (ADA), are as follows:

- fasting blood sugar level ≥* 126 mg/dL (7.0 mmol/L)

- at two hours in the Oral Glucose Tolerance Test (OGTT; see below), blood sugar level ≥200 mg/dL (11.1 mmol/L)

- random blood sugar ≥200 mg/dL (11.1 mmol/L) and symptoms of diabetes

- HbA1c ≥6.5 percent (48 mmol/mol)

Table 1 compares the normal, pre-diabetic, and diabetic ranges of both blood sugar and HbA1c values.

Oral Glucose Tolerance Test (OGTT)

A commonly used diagnostic test for type 2 diabetes is called the two hour **oral glucose tolerance test (OGTT)**. This is done after fasting (no food for at least 8 hours). First, a fasting blood sugar (glucose) sample is drawn; then the person drinks a high sugar drink (e.g., Glucola™) within five minutes. A second blood sugar sample is drawn after two hours. Many people get diagnosed with diabetes because of an abnormally high blood sugar level after two hours, even though their fasting blood sugar level is normal. Diabetes is diagnosed if either the fasting blood sugar is ≥126 mg/dL (7.0 mmol/L) or the two hour blood sugar is ≥200 mg/dL (11.1 mmol/L).

*≥ This symbol represents "greater than or equal to."

TABLE 1

Oral Glucose Tolerance Test (OGTT), Blood Sugar Values and HbA1c Values

Blood Sugar	Normal		Pre-Diabetes		Diabetes	
	mg/dL	mmol/L	mg/dL	mmol/L	mg/dL	mmol/L
Fasting	<100	<5.5*	100-125	5.5-6.9	≥126*	≥7.0
2 hours after drinking the sugar-load	<140	<7.8	140-200	7.8-11.0	≥200	≥11.1
HbA1c						
percent	<6		5.7-6.4		≥6.5	
mmol/mol	<42		39-46		≥48	

* < = Symbol for "less-than;" ≥ = symbol for "greater-than or equal to."

FIGURE 2

Formation of HbA1c from Hemoglobin and Sugar

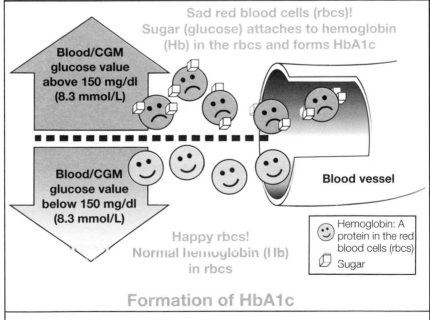

Formation of HbA1c

The hemoglobin A1c (hemoglobin+ attached sugar) reflects the average blood sugar every second of the day for the past three months. HbA1c values are higher when sugar levels have been higher.

Hemoglobin A1c (HbA1c, A1c)

Another diagnostic test is the hemoglobin A1c level (HbA1c, or A1c). Sugar in the blood stream attaches to the hemoglobin molecules in red blood cells (see Figure 2) which is what this test measures. Thus, with higher blood sugar levels, the HbA1c value rises. It reflects the average blood sugar level over the previous three months. The HbA1c level for people without diabetes is usually below 6.0 percent (42 mmol/mol). The ADA considers a value above 6.5 percent (46 mmol/mol) to be diagnostic of diabetes.

People with diabetes should know what the HbA1c level represents, know their last value, and know how they can improve the level (if needed). After the diagnosis of diabetes has been made, the HbA1c level should be measured every three to six months if adequately controlled (below 7.0 percent or 53 mmol/mol) or every three months if above that level.

More recently, some groups consider the HbA1c level to be more accurate than blood sugar values as a means to diagnose pre-diabetes and diabetes. The OGTT and the fasting blood sugar level are more difficult to perform, reflect only that moment in time, and may not be as reliable.

SUMMARY

Type 2 diabetes is caused by a combination of factors including an inherited genetic risk and an unhealthy lifestyle that promotes obesity and insulin resistance. High calorie diets and lack of exercise may cause a gradual progression of insulin resistance, resulting in high blood sugar levels that could go on for years before symptoms appear. Type 2 diabetes may be suspected using a combination of factors such as family history, classic symptoms (see above), blood sugar levels, HbA1c level or other parameters. It is critical to make the diagnosis so treatment can begin and complications can be prevented.

BASIC NUTRITION

Dena Gottesman, MS, RD, CDE, H. Peter Chase, MD,
Satish K. Garg, MD

U nderstanding basic nutrition is a skill everyone can benefit from, but is especially important for those who have diabetes or who are at risk for diabetes.

CALORIES

Energy from food is measured in calories. The three types of food providing energy are:
- carbohydrates
- proteins
- fats

Proteins and carbohydrates provide four calories for each gram of food eaten. Fat provides nine calories for each gram of food eaten. Thus, eating foods higher in fat often leads to greater weight gain. When not using calories, such as when not doing regular exercise, the unused energy gets stored in the body as fat. Reduction of total caloric intake is usually required for weight loss. Reducing portion sizes of food results in a reduction of caloric intake. Using a smaller plate for meals and avoiding high fat foods, second-helpings and snacks may also help to reduce caloric intake. Balancing the intake of these nutrients in your diet can help lead to successful diabetes management. Maintaining a healthy body weight is an important factor in managing diabetes.

CARBOHYDRATES

Carbohydrates are our main source of energy and are the primary food that affects blood sugar levels. All carbohydrates are converted to sugar and are absorbed in the small intestine. However, different kinds of carbohydrates are absorbed at different speeds and are utilized differently. Simple carbohydrates pass through the stomach quickly for absorption in the intestine. Some examples of simple carbohydrates are high-sugar drinks (e.g., soda and juice), which should be avoided by people with diabetes unless needed to treat a low blood sugar.

Complex carbohydrates (e.g., fruits, vegetables and whole grains) must first be broken down in the stomach before arriving in the small intestine. This longer journey allows for slower absorption of the sugar, affecting the blood sugar more slowly. This makes complex carbohydrates better choices for people with diabetes. The current recommendation is to eat at least five servings per day of fruits and vegetables. Because all carbohydrates are broken down into sugar, it is essential that people with diabetes be aware of and keep track of all carbohydrate intake. Understanding how carbohydrates affect your blood sugar levels empowers you to make healthy food choices.

FIBER

Dietary fiber is the part of plants not digested or absorbed into the body. It's often known as "roughage" or "bulk." There are two types of fiber: water-soluble fibers and insoluble fibers. Water-soluble fibers are found in oats, beans, lentils and seeds, as well as in some fruits like citrus fruits, apples and pears. These soluble fiber foods may help to lower cholesterol and LDL-cholesterol levels. Intake of one cup per day of legumes (e.g., cooked beans, chick peas or lentils) has been shown to lower HbA1c levels by approximately 0.5 percent (5 mmol/mol). In general, it seems that in most studies the intake of fiber had to be very high (44-50 grams/day) to improve glycemic (sugar) control. This is unlikely to be adhered to over a prolonged period. However, it is a good idea to strive to eat high-fiber foods. The U.S. Department of Agriculture recommends eating 14 grams of fiber for every 1,000 calories consumed. Intake of whole grain foods is also encouraged.

Carbohydrates high in fiber generally do not raise blood sugar levels as much as do foods low in fiber. They are referred to as having a low "**glycemic index**." However, several studies have not found differences in HbA1c levels for people consuming a high glycemic index diet compared to a low glycemic index diet. Thus, the ADA no longer makes nutritional recommendations for diabetes management based on glycemic index.

PROTEIN

Most Americans eat more protein than the current dietary guidelines recommend. Foods high in protein, for example, include meats, beans and cheeses. Muscle is built by exercising, not by eating extra protein. Increased protein intake can be stressful on the kidneys. Since kidneys can be affected by diabetes (see Chapter 16), people with diabetes should aim for normal protein intake. The current recommendation is for 20 percent of calories to be from protein, 30 percent from fat, and 50 percent from carbohydrate. It is important for a meal to have a balance of carbohydrates, protein and fat. This combination helps to slow the absorption of carbohydrates, and thus slow the rise of blood sugar levels.

FAT

As noted above, fat has more than twice the calories of carbohydrates and proteins. Reducing fat intake is an important component in a weight loss program. There are several types of fats, including monounsaturated and polyunsaturated fats (generally considered "healthy" fats) and the saturated and trans fats (considered "unhealthy" fats). Polyunsaturated fats include most vegetable oils (corn, safflower, soy, sunflower) and olive oil. Foods higher in saturated fat include the following:

- red meats
- the skin of chicken or turkey
- whole milk and dairy products
- fats and oils (e.g., butter, margarine, mayonnaise, etc.)

Portions of the fats found in the bloodstream (e.g., cholesterol and triglycerides) come from fat in the diet. Higher levels are usually related to cardiovascular (heart and blood vessel) disease. Adults with diabetes are at greater risk for cardiovascular disease, making it even more important to reduce their fat intake. Recommendations for blood lipid levels are provided in Table 1.

TABLE 1

Recommended Levels for Lipids and Lipoproteins

Lipid Type	Desired Level**	
Cholesterol	< 200 mg/dL	< 5.2 mmol/L
LDL Cholesterol*	< 100 mg/dL	< 2.6 mmol/L
HDL Cholesterol*	> 40 mg/dL	> 1.0 mmol/L
Triglyceride*	< 150 mg/dL	< 1.7 mmol/L

*Preferably drawn after fasting overnight. If fasting overnight is not possible, then at least four hours after eating.

**Desired level for a person with diabetes

**< equals less than; > equals greater than

SODIUM

Salt in the diet plays a large role in maintaining a person's blood pressure. Some people are more sensitive to salt intake than others. People with elevated blood pressure generally need to restrict salt in their diet. Be mindful that table salt is not the only culprit of high salt content in foods. Salt is often hidden in packaged and processed foods. The American Heart Association recommends all people limit their sodium to less than 1500 mg (3/4 teaspoon) per day. The amount should be even lower if the blood pressure is elevated. Elevated blood pressure can lead to cardiovascular disease, which is more common in adults with diabetes. Reading food labels (Table 2) and watching sodium intake are helpful in making healthier food choices.

OTHER NUTRIENTS

Vitamins and minerals (especially calcium) are also important. They are discussed in the book, *Understanding Diabetes,*

SWEETENERS

Sweeteners are divided into "nutritive" and "non-nutritive." The nutritive sweeteners (including table sugar) provide carbohydrate calories and may raise blood sugar levels. High-fructose corn syrup is now added to many foods and many physicians consider this sugar more harmful than plain table sugar.

The non-nutritive (or "artificial") sweeteners (e.g., saccharin, aspartame, acesulfame-potassium, sucrolose, stevia, etc.) have helped people with diabetes avoid high blood sugar levels. However, some studies have shown that even drinking diet sodas leads to increased weight gain. The reason is not yet known.

LIQUIDS

Water is the best liquid to drink. Water makes up approximately 80 percent of our body. It is lost throughout the day and must be replaced. Everyone should drink four to eight glasses of water per day. Drinking a glass of water for rehydration first thing in the morning is wise.

Some studies have found drinking coffee or tea reduces the risk for developing type 2 diabetes. It is important to remember that adding cream, milk and/or sugar increases the calorie content of the drink. Drinking regular (sugar) soda has been shown to relate to insulin resistance, which is a big part of type 2 diabetes. People with diabetes, or who are at risk for developing diabetes, should NOT consume regular (sugar) pop (other than to treat low blood sugar).

ALCOHOL

Many alcoholic drinks, including beer, are high in sugar and can cause a rise in blood sugar levels initially. However, blood sugars may become low up to 12 hours later, particularly in people taking medications such as sulfonylureas or insulin. This is because alcohol reduces sugar production from the liver. A small snack composed of complex carbohydrate, protein and fat and not "sleeping-in" the morning after alcohol consumption may be helpful in preventing a low blood sugar.

READING A FOOD LABEL

The U.S. law requires labeling of the nutritional content of food products. Smart consumers can learn a lot about the foods to purchase by being savvy label readers. The information gained from reading a food label is discussed in Table 2.

The carbohydrate grams are listed under "total carbohydrate" on most labels. This value usually includes the grams of dietary fiber, which are absorbed more slowly, if at all. Determining the grams of carbohydrate in a food item is essential for a carbohydrate counting food plan (see Chapter 4). It is also important, especially for weight loss, to read the total fat content on the nutrition label.

3-DAY FOOD RECORD

It is often helpful for the dietitian to have a 3-day record of what you've been eating and drinking. If you do this (See Table 3), it is important to be honest and to eat as you normally do. This will provide valuable information to help manage your diabetes.

SUMMARY

In summary, eating healthy, balanced and nutritious meals and snacks can be helpful for all family members. The ideal food plan for a person with diabetes is a healthy diet from which most people would benefit.

TABLE 2
Reading a Food Label

- The serving size is shown at the top. It is important to observe the serving size. (This is often less than the amount people eat. If you eat two cups rather than one, you would need to double all of the amounts listed.) The total calories and the calories from fat per serving are routinely given and are important.

- The total fat includes all types of fat (saturated, polyunsaturated, monounsaturated and trans-fat). The total fat, saturated fat and cholesterol content are all important in relation to heart disease and it is wise to look for lower fat choices.

- The saturated fats for the entire day should be under 10 percent of the total calories per day. For someone eating 2,000 calories per day, this would mean under 200 calories from saturated fat or under 22g (nine calories per gram). The trans-fat content appears on the label as of 2006.

- †The percent of daily values for fat, carbohydrate and protein are listed on the label based on a 2,000 calorie daily intake. More active people will need more calories, in which case these amounts should be figured based on calories actually eaten.

Nutrition Facts	
Serving Size 1.0 Cup (120g)	
Servings Per Container	8

Amount Per Serving	
Calories 130 Calories From Fat 60	
	% Daily Value †
Total Fat 6.5g	10%
Saturated Fat 2.5g	12%
Trans-fat	0%
Cholesterol 30mg	10%
Sodium 240mg	10%
Total Carbohydrate 15g	5%
Dietary Fiber 2.5g	10%
Sugars 3g	
Protein 3g	6%
Vitamin A 10% Vitamin E 5%	
Calcium 15% Iron 5%	

†Percent Daily Values are based on a 2,000-calorie diet. Your daily values may be higher or lower depending on your calorie needs:

Calories:	2,000	2,500	3,200
Total Fat (g)	65	80	107
Sat Fat (g)	20	25	36
Cholesterol (mg)	300	300	300
Sodium (mg)	2,400	2,400	2,400
Total Carb (g)	300	375	480
Fiber	25	30	37

Calories per gram:
Fat 9   Carbohydrate 4   Protein 4

Ingredients: Whole wheat, oat bran, raisins, gelatin, malt, flavoring, vitamins, and minerals.

- For those who count carbohydrates, one helping of this cereal has 15g of carbohydrate, which is one carbohydrate exchange. If one cup of white milk (any type) is added, then one additional carbohydrate exchange must also be added so that there would be a total of two carbohydrate exchanges. The sugars include those found naturally in the food as well as those added to the food. Both are included in the grams of "Total Carbohydrate."

- The recommended daily amounts for cholesterol stay the same for the 24-hour period for the three caloric intakes.

- The ingredients on the example are usually included on the label in order of the amount present.

TABLE 3

Three-Day Food Record Form

Instructions for completing food record form:

1. Please write down everything you eat or drink for three days. This includes meals and snacks. Often it's easier to remember what you eat if you record your food intake at the time you eat it.

2. Include the amount (portion size) of food or beverage eaten. Also note the method of preparation (baked, fried, broiled, etc.), as well as any brand names of products (labels can also be enclosed). Use standard measuring cups or spoons. Measure the meat portions in ounces after cooking. If you do not have a scale, you can estimate ounces. The size of a deck of cards is about equal to three ounces of meat.

3. Be sure to include items added to your food, like condiments or sauces (e.g., salad dressing, dips, butter or margarine, or ketchup).

4. Include any supplements you take (vitamin, mineral or protein powders). Write down the name of the supplement, what it contains and the amount taken. Include a copy of the label, if possible.

5. Please include meal and snack times, blood glucose values, amount and type of insulin, type of food, amount of food, grams of carbohydrate and any activity or exercise. Put a star next to any blood sugar value that is two hours after a meal.

The following is an example of how to complete your food record. Please record what you eat on the forms in this chapter. The forms can then be faxed or mailed to your diabetes care-provider. *An example for the start of a day follows:*

Time	Blood Glucose	Insulin	Food (include amounts)	Carbs	Activity
8:00	170	4H/10N	Cheerios-= 1 1/2 Cup	34g	
			Fat free milk- 1 cup	12g	
10:00					Jog - 20 min

3-DAY FOOD RECORD
(copy as needed)

Name: _____

Date: _____

Dietitian: _____

Home #: _____

Cell or Work #: _____

Best time to be reached _____

Insulin-to-Carb ratios (if known)

Breakfast: _____

Lunch: _____

Dinner: _____

Snack: _____

Blood Sugar Correction:

_____

Time	Blood Glucose	Insulin	Food (include amounts)	Carbs	Activity

DIABETES AND FOOD MANAGEMENT

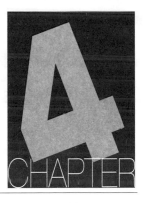

Dona Gottesman, MS, RD, CDE, H. Peter Chase, MD,
Satish K. Garg, MD

Meeting with a dietitian to learn about nutrition, types of foods and a food plan is important for people newly diagnosed with either type 1 or type 2 diabetes. Although food management is a vital component for both types of diabetes, achieving weight loss is often a much greater priority for people with type 2 diabetes.

Obesity is commonly regarded as a primary cause of insulin resistance. The combination of reduced intake of calories along with regular exercise is the most effective way to achieve weight loss. Weight loss and/or weight management is a key goal for the majority of people with type 2 diabetes. Losing weight is equally important for those with pre-type 2 diabetes to prevent and/or delay the onset of type 2 diabetes.

GENERAL PRINCIPLES FOR HEALTHY NUTRITION

- Maintain a healthy weight.
- Eat well-balanced meals and snacks throughout the day.
- Eat foods with fewer calories and smaller portion sizes.
- Avoid concentrated sweets (e.g., regular sugar soda, fruit juice - which includes 100 percent juice and no sugar added juices, and pure sugar candies and sweets).
- Reduce saturated fat content of meals and snacks.
- Eat 20-35 grams of fiber daily, including non-starchy vegetables and whole grains. Fruits and vegetables should add up to at least five servings per day.
- Limit unhealthy choices, such as fried foods, and fast foods (e.g., burgers, fries, pizza).
- Avoid consuming excess and/or "empty" calories.
- Choose fewer foods that are high in salt (sodium).
- If consuming alcohol, do so in moderation.
- Choose lean meat (for protein).

19

If applicable, learn to adjust insulin doses. In other words, decrease dose for exercise or alcohol intake, or increase dose with infections, menses or with a reduction in exercise (such as a trip in a car).

FOOD PLANS

Weight Management

Weight loss only occurs if there is a negative energy balance. This can happen with reduced caloric intake or with increased burning of calories through exercise. Most every food plan that involves reducing caloric intake will provide weight loss if the person is motivated to stick to it. It is important to find a food plan that the person likes and will adhere to and follow. After initial weight loss, there is often a "leveling-off" of the effect. This is normal and the person must still follow the plan and not become discouraged. Exercise may need to be increased to one hour per day, six days per week, in addition to following the food plan.

Unfortunately, there is no "one-size-fits-all" food plan to achieve weight loss or weight maintenance. Weight loss has been successful with various types of food plans, including a low-fat, low-carbohydrate, calorie restricted meal plan or a Mediterranean-style food plan. The Mediterranean food plan recommends high intake of fresh fruits and vegetables, with fish, beans and nuts as a protein source (whole eggs limited to once weekly, egg whites more frequently and red meat once or twice monthly). Whole grains are recommended as a major source of carbohydrate. Consider soups and salads and home-prepared nutritious meals! A website to learn more about the Mediterranean food plan is http://www.mediterraneanbook.com/the-mediterranean-diet/. An additional resource is from the Academy of Nutrition and Dietetics, http://www.eatright.org. It can also be helpful to meet with a dietitian who will be able to provide the proper guidance to determine what's best for you.

Glucose (Sugar) Management

Most people with type 1 diabetes follow a food plan. The primary focus is on carbohydrate management rather than weight loss. The two food plans below may also be helpful for people with type 2 diabetes when treated with insulin. There are two types of food plans most commonly used when taking insulin, **Constant Carbohydrate** and **Carbohydrate Counting**.

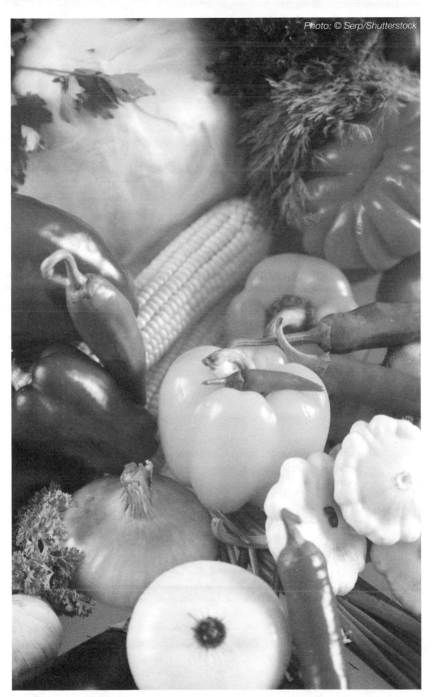

The Mediterranean food plan recommends high intake of fresh fruits and vegetables. The current recommendation is for all people to eat at least five servings per day of fruits and vegetables.

Constant Carbohydrate

- This plan involves eating a consistent amount of carbohydrate grams for each meal and for each snack throughout each day. Insulin doses are adjusted based on the blood sugar level and other factors such as exercise, illness, stress, menses, etc.

A ***Carbohydrate ("Carb") Counting*** food plan is often used once the person has a better understanding of how carbohydrates impact the blood sugar level.

- This plan involves counting the carbohydrate grams of food to be consumed. If on insulin, then determine the appropriate dose of rapid-acting insulin to match the carbohydrates. The formula to calculate the dose is called an insulin-to-carb ratio or "I/C ratio."
- The dietitian may want a three-day diet record to be done before the I/C ratio is determined (see Chapter 3). The healthcare team and family choose an I/C ratio. A common ratio often used when starting this plan is one unit of insulin for each 15 grams of carbohydrate (I/C ratio of 1 unit to 15 grams).
- Gradually, the correct ratios for each meal are determined. The I/C ratio may vary for each meal of the day.

To test the accuracy of an I/C ratio, blood sugar levels are checked two hours after a meal and before the next meal.

- If the blood sugar level is high (e.g., over 180 mg/dL or 10.0 mmol/L), the I/C ratio could be changed from 1 unit to 15 grams to 1 unit to 12 (or even 10) grams of carbohydrates.
- If the blood sugar level is low (e.g., less than 70 mg/dL or 3.6 mmol/L), the I/C ratio could be changed to 1 unit to 20 grams of carbs.
- If a pre-meal blood sugar level is high, an additional amount of insulin may be needed (a "correction" dose; see Chapter 11). The correction dose is then added to the I/C ratio dose. Together, this will be the total dose of insulin given before the meal or snack. Adjustment of the basal insulin dose (Chapter 7) may also be needed.
- If blood sugar levels are above the desired upper level one to two hours after a meal and the pre-meal blood sugar is above 90 mg/dL or 5.0 mmol/L, it may be beneficial to give the rapid-acting insulin 15 to 20 minutes before the meal. This technique works because blood sugar levels usually peak in 60 minutes after a meal, whereas rapid-acting insulins (Chapter 7) do not peak until 90-100 minutes after injection.

TABLE 1
Sugar Content of Some High-Carbohydrate Foods

Food Item	Size Portion	Sugar Content* teaspoons)	"Carb" Choices	Gram Carb
Beverage				
Cola drinks	12 oz can	10	3	50
Root beer	12 oz can	7	2	35
7-Up®*	12 oz can	9	3	45
Grape, orange, apple juice	6 oz can	5	1½	25
Dairy Products				
Sherbet	1 scoop	9	3	45
Ice cream cone	1 scoop	3½	1	17
Chocolate milk shake	10 oz glass	11	4	55
Milk	8 oz glass	3	1	12
Chocolate milk	8 oz glass	9½	3	52
Fruit yogurt	8 oz cup	9	3	45
Cakes and Cookies				
Angel food cake	4 oz piece	7	2	35
Chocolate cake, plain	4 oz piece	6	2	30
Chocolate cake, w/frosting	4 oz piece	10	3	50
Sugar cookie	1	1½	½	7
Oatmeal cookie	1	2	1	10
Donut, plain	1	4	1	20
Donut, glazed	1	6	2	30
Desserts				
JELL-O	½ cup	4½	1½	22
Apple pie	1 slice	7	2	35
Berry pie	1 slice	10	3	50
Chocolate pudding	½ cup	4	1	20
Candies				
Chocolate candy bar	1½ oz	2½	1	12
Chewing gum	1 stick	½	-	2
Fudge	1 oz square	4½	1½	22
Hard candy	1 oz	5	2	25
LIFE-SAVERS®	1	⅓	-	1½
Marshmallow	1 piece	1½	½	7
Chocolate creme	1 piece	2	1	10
Miscellaneous				
Jelly	1 Tbsp	3	1	15
Strawberry jam	1 Tbsp	3	1	15
Brown sugar	1 Tbsp	3	1	15
Honey	1 Tbsp	3	1	15
Chocolate sauce	1 Tbsp	3	1	15
Karo Syrup®	1 Tbsp	3	1	15

*3 tsp = 1 Tbsp = 1 carb choice = 15g of carbs

From: *Understanding Diabetes*, 12th Ed., p 120

Table 1 gives the carbohydrate content of some high-carbohydrate foods. Intake of these foods should be limited in people with diabetes.

To quote a well respected dietitian:*"Nutrition therapy for diabetes mellitus is effective. However, just as there is no one medication or insulin regimen appropriate for all persons with diabetes mellitus, there is no one nutrition therapy intervention. A variety of nutrition therapy interventions have been shown to be effective. Nutrition education and counseling must be sensitive to the personal needs and cultural preferences of individuals and their ability to make and sustain lifestyle changes."

SUMMARY

It is recommended that all people with diabetes follow a food plan. Food management is crucial for people with type 2 diabetes, especially when focusing on weight loss and/or weight control. Additionally, large quantities of concentrated sweets should be avoided by everyone with diabetes.

*Marion J. Franz, MS, RD, CDE, Arch Intern Med 172, 1660, 2012

EXERCISE AND DIABETES

R egular exercise is important for everyone. However, it is even more important for people with diabetes. A healthy lifestyle, consisting of regular exercise and wholesome eating, is essential for weight control in people with type 2 and type 1 diabetes.

Exercise can also help to prevent type 2 diabetes. An important study* found that people with pre-type 2 diabetes were less likely to progress to diabetes if they made healthy lifestyle changes with a modest weight loss. This included at least 150 minutes of moderate exercise (e.g., brisk walking) per week along with a healthy low calorie, low fat weight loss program resulting in a body weight reduction of at least 7 percent. More recent evidence suggests that 60 minutes of exercise at least six days per week is necessary for weight loss and maintenance.

EXERCISE & TYPE 2 DIABETES

For people with type 2 diabetes, exercise, along with reduced caloric intake, is essential for weight loss management. Exercise is one of the "big four" factors that affect blood sugar levels—along with medications, food, and stress (see Figure 1). It also has the unique benefit of making a person's body more sensitive to insulin. This means the body will need less insulin to use sugar and the pancreas will not have to work as hard to produce large amounts of insulin. Exercise is one of the main behavioral changes that can help address the underlying problems in people with type 2 diabetes.

If people with type 2 diabetes exercise regularly and lose weight, they may be able to reduce or stop their oral medications. This should only be attempted if agreed to by a healthcare-provider. Table 1 summarizes some of the reasons why exercise is important.

*Diabetes Prevention Program, N Engl J Med 246, 393, 2002

TABLE 1

Why Exercise is Important

- Exercise lowers blood sugar levels.
- Exercise helps people feel better.
- Exercise helps maintain proper body weight.
- Exercise helps lower the heart rate (pulse) and blood pressure.
- Exercise helps keep blood fat levels normal.
- Exercise improves insulin sensitivity.
- Exercise may help maintain normal blood circulation in the feet.

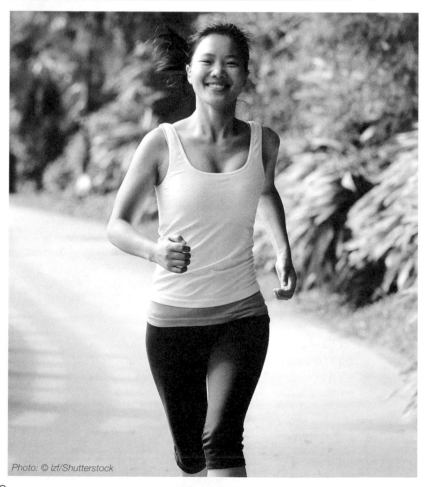

Photo: © Izf/Shutterstock

FIGURE 1

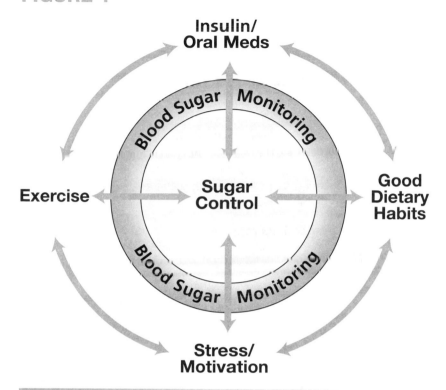

Four of the Major Influences on Blood Sugar Control.

All four must be in balance for the best sugar control. Blood sugar control is measured by daily blood/CGM levels and by Hemoglobin A1C (HbA1c) levels done every three months.

A few key points about exercise and diabetes are summarized below.

- Exercise is **essential** for weight control and general health.

- Exercise is one of the "big four" factors, along with medications, food, and stress which affect blood sugar levels (see Figure 1).

- Exercise can lower blood sugar levels and help keep them in the target range. It does this in part by making people more sensitive to insulin (see Figure 2).

- The type of exercise can be varied depending on personal interests and goals (e.g., weight loss or muscle build-up). Calories expended for various activities are shown in Table 2.

- **The usual recommendation for daily activity is for at least 30 to 60 minutes every day.**

- It is important to drink extra water during strenuous exercise to prevent dehydration.

PREVENTING LOW BLOOD SUGARS (HYPOGLYCEMIA)

Low blood sugar levels can occur with exercise because it makes the body more sensitive to insulin. The muscle cells also burn more sugar with exercise than resting. Exercise can cause the blood sugar levels to become low. This occurs most frequently with people taking insulin or sulfonylurea medications (see Chapter 6).

The following suggestions may help to prevent low blood sugars (some suggestions apply only to people who check blood sugar levels).

- If hypoglycemia happens frequently with exercise, discuss changes in your medication dosages with your doctor.

- Always carry a source of fast-acting carbohydrate (e.g., glucose tablets or glucose gel) when exercising.

- Check blood sugar levels more frequently before, during, and after exercise.

- Make sure your diabetes healthcare-provider downloads your glucose meter during your clinic visits and knows the days and times of exercise.

- Keep a log of blood sugar levels when starting exercise or increasing time or effort. This will help with management in the future.

- Aim for a slightly higher blood sugar level before exercise (160-180 mg/dL [8.9-10.0 mmol/L]).

- Consume extra snacks as needed before, during, and after exercise. Use about 4 ounces of drinks such as Gatorade® every 30 minutes during intense exercise.

- If hypoglycemia happens during exercise (below 70 mg/dL or 3.9 mmol/L), stop exercising and consume 15g of fast-acting carbohydrates. Do not resume exercise until the blood sugar level is above 90 mg/dL or 5.0 mmol/L. The "rule of 15" is to consume 15 grams of sugar and to recheck the blood sugar level in 15 minutes.

- Add an extra 15 or 30 grams of carbohydrate at bedtime if afternoon or evening exercise was strenuous.

- If taking basal insulin, talk to your diabetes care-provider about how to safely reduce insulin to avoid low blood sugar levels.

- If checking blood sugar levels, make sure the bedtime level is above 130 mg/dL (7.2 mmol/L) on exercise days. Wake up in the middle of the night to check your level when starting or changing the exercise routine.

HYDRATION AND EXERCISE

Proper hydration (drinking fluids) is essential during exercise. Exercising during hot weather requires special attention. There is a higher risk of heat stroke and dehydration, so extra fluids are recommended. Drinking extra fluids should begin an hour or two before starting to exercise. A general rule is to drink eight ounces of fluids for every 30 minutes of vigorous activity.

Liquids such as sports drinks (e.g., Gatorade) help replace water, salts and carbohydrates. Drinking sports drinks at 30 minute intervals in conjunction with blood sugar checking (if taking insulin) during strenuous exercise works well in avoiding low blood sugars. However, sports drinks should be consumed in moderation. Some people dilute 4-8 ounces of a sports drink in water. The dilution depends on the exercise effort and if more fluid is needed. This will decrease the carbohydrate intake while maintaining hydration.

BEGINNING AN EXERCISE PROGRAM

Adults are advised to discuss plans to begin a new exercise program with their physician first. It is important to start slowly and gradually increase the amount of exercise. Proper stretching (five to 10 minutes) BEFORE, DURING and AFTER the exercise will help to prevent cramps and stiffness that may otherwise discourage further exercise.

If using insulin, your dose may need to be reduced when starting exercise. Any changes will need to be fine-tuned for your weight, effort and length of time of exercise. This should be discussed with a diabetes healthcare-provider.

Having a medical check-up before starting a new exercise program is recommended for people who:

- are over 35 years of age

- have had type 1 diabetes for more than 15 years

- have additional risk factors for a heart attack

- have eye or kidney complications

- have neuropathy (Chapter 16)

A graded exercise test might also be helpful. The maximum heart rate during exercise should not exceed 220 minus age.

Strenuous activities, including weight lifting and jogging, are discouraged for people who have the severe eye changes of diabetes (proliferative retinopathy). The extra pressure can increase the likelihood of further eye problems. This should be discussed with the diabetes eye specialist. Similarly, people with neuropathy should discuss the pros and cons of exercise with their physician. When peripheral neuropathy is severe, weight-bearing exercises should be limited. With both severe eye changes and neuropathy, exercise that involves straining, jarring or increased pressure on the eyes or feet must be avoided.

It is sometimes wise to have a baseline electrocardiogram (EKG) done prior to beginning a new exercise program. Further evaluation is then possible if there are any suggestions of abnormalities. You may ask your diabetes healthcare-provider to review the ADA guidelines for exercise with you (published in the annual January Supplement to "Diabetes Care").

SUMMARY

Exercise is a major part of living a healthy lifestyle, especially for people with diabetes. Oral medications and insulin dose (if taking insulin) may need to be adjusted to avoid low blood sugars. Always keep fast-acting sugar (glucose) nearby and drink plenty of fluids. Check with your diabetes care team about possible complications or limiting factors. Most importantly, try to exercise daily!

TABLE 2

Calories Burned Per Hour In Common Physical Activities

Moderate Physical Activity for One Hour	Calories Burned Per Hour
Hiking	370
Light gardening/yard work	330
Dancing	330
Golf (walking and carrying clubs)	330
Bicycling (<10 mph)	290
Walking (3.5 mph)	280
Weight lifting (general light workout)	220
Stretching	180
Vigorous Physical Activity for One Hour:	
Running/jogging (5 mph)	590
Bicycling (>10 mph)	590
Swimming (slow freestyle laps)	510
Aerobics	480
Walking (4.5 mph)	460
Heavy yard work (chopping wood)	440
Weight lifting (vigorous effort)	440
Basketball (vigorous)	440

*Source: Adapted from the 2005 "DGAC Report" and the
"Dietary Guidelines for Americans", 2005*

FIGURE 2

Blood Sugars With and Without One Hour of Exercise

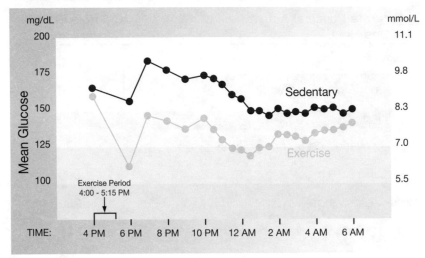

This figure represents blood sugar levels for the same 50 people on a sedentary day (black circles) and an exercise day blue circles). The one hour of exercise at 4 p.m. resulted in lower blood sugar levels for the next 14 hours (through the night). Insulin doses and food intake were identical for the two days.

Data compliments of the DirecNet Study Group: J Pediatr 147,528, 2005

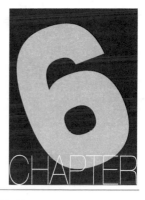

TYPE 2 DIABETES MEDICATIONS

TREATMENT OPTIONS FOR TYPE 2 DIABETES

The choice of treatment for type 2 diabetes varies with different providers. It is usually a step-wise approach that starts with minimal intervention and changes are then made as needed (see Figure 1). Several possible steps, or "stages" of therapy, as used in our Center, are outlined below. Some of the considerations that go into choosing a therapy are as follows:

- the individual's motivation to take care of him/herself
- whether the individual is able to monitor blood sugar levels adequately
- safety (especially the prevention of low blood sugars)
- how well each medication will control blood sugar levels
- how well each medication will prevent complications of diabetes
- financial situation
- other factors (e.g., providers' comfort level with a given medication)

It is important that the treatment regimen is individualized as needed. No matter what stage of treatment is selected, healthy living is essential for all stages. This includes making healthy food choices and daily exercise (as discussed in Chapters 2-5). The stages below are listed in an order frequently used at our Center.

STAGE 1: HEALTHY LIFESTYLE

All people with type 2 diabetes are advised to change their lifestyle as a first step in their treatment. Living a healthy lifestyle may be all that is needed in the initial stage of treatment of type 2 diabetes. Healthy living includes making wise food choices as well as daily exercise. Healthy food choices include eating more fruits, vegetables and whole grains and eliminating frequent consumption of foods high in sugar or fat (see Chapter 4). Portion sizes also need to be reduced. Blood sugar monitoring may not be needed at this early stage of type 2 diabetes management. Modest weight loss results in excellent outcomes.

FIGURE 1

Treatment Stages for Type 2 Diabetes*

Stage 1:
Healthy lifestyle

⬇

Stage 2:
Add metformin

⬇

Stage 3: Add a second oral medication or (injectable) basal insulin or GLP-1 analog:

- DPP-4 inhibitors: sitagliptin (Januvia), saxagliptin (Onglyza), linagliptin (Trajenta), vidagliptin (Galvus) and alogliptin (Nesina).

- Other medications like thiozolidinediones (Actos®), -Glucosidase inhibitors (Acarbose®), meglitinides (Repaglinide®, Nateglinide®), etc.

- Basal insulin: NPH, glargine (Lantus), detemir (Levemir), degludec (Tresiba)

- GLP-1 analogs: exenatide (Byetta), exenatide extended release (Bydureon), or liraglutide (Victoza)

Stage 4:
- Add basal insulin: NPH, glargine (Lantus), detemir (Levemir), or degludec (Tresiba)

Stage 5:
Using a combination of a basal insulin and a GLP-1 analog

Stage 6:
Add meal-time insulin: lispro (Humalog), aspart (Novolog), or glulisine (Aprida)

Some of these medicines are "complex." You only need to read about the medicine you are receiving.

STAGE 2: METFORMIN

When people are not able to achieve the desired glucose control as measured by HbA1c level (e.g., below 7.0 percent or 53 mmol/mol) with a healthy lifestyle alone, metformin is usually added to the treatment regime. Metformin works by decreasing the amount of sugar that the liver produces. At this stage, occasional blood sugar monitoring is often recommended. For example, 4-6 blood sugar checks in one day every 2-3 months may be advised. The 4-6 blood sugar checks in one day might include fasting, before and/or two hours after meals and before bed. Metformin, when used alone, does not cause low blood sugar problems. The blood sugar checks are to make sure the dose of metformin is controlling the blood sugar levels. Table 1 summarizes administration, action and side-effects of the type 2 medications most frequently used in our clinic.

STAGE 3: ADDITION OF OTHER MEDICINES

This option is considered particularly if blood sugar levels and the HbA1c values are not improved within three to six months on metformin. If metformin does not achieve the target HbA1c level (e.g., below 7.0 percent or 53 mmol/L), a second medication is usually added. As noted below, some physicians add insulin or other oral medicines early during Stage 2. Different choices for a second medicine are outlined below.

- **DPP4-Inhibitors:**
  Glucagon-like poly-peptide (GLP-1) is a normal protein in the body that works by increasing the person's own insulin secretion as needed, decreasing glucagon levels after meals, delaying stomach emptying, and decreasing appetite (all helpful). Unfortunately, GLP-1 levels are reduced in people with type 2 diabetes. Oral medicines have been developed that prevent GLP-1 breakdown, thus raising GLP-1 levels. These medicines are called dipeptidyl peptidase-4 inhibitors (DPP-4 inhibitors). Examples of DPP-4 inhibitor medicines are sitagliptin (Januvia®), saxagliptin (Onglyza®), linagliptin (Trajenta®), vidagliptin (Galvuls®) and alogliptin (Nesina®). The DPP-4 inhibitors or the GLP-1 analogs (see below) may be helpful as a second medicine (with metformin). The DPP-4 inhibitors result in modest improvements in HbA1c levels.

- **GLP-1 Analogs (GLP-1 receptor agonists):**
  Medications (analogs) that mimic (also called "GLP-1 mimetics") Glucagon-like poly-peptide (GLP-1) action have also been developed. Examples of GLP-1 analog medicines include exenatide (Byetta®), exenatide extended release (Bydureon®),

liraglutide (Victoza®) and lixisenatide (Lyxuma®) (only available in Europe). These medications only come in injectable form. Use of the GLP-1 analogs can result in significant drops in the HbA1c levels.

It is important to be aware of possible side effects. The GLP-1 analogs may cause nausea, vomiting and diarrhea in 30 to 40 percent of people. To avoid or reduce these side effects, it is important to start with a small dose and gradually build up to a tolerable dose. Some people may not be able to tolerate these medications at all. Also, two other important, but rare, side effects listed by the FDA include risk of pancreatitis and 'c-cell' hyperplasia in the thyroid gland. The long term effects of these medications are not known. If tolerated, most patients lose weight.

With either the DDP-4 inhibitors or the GLP-1 analogs, the frequency of blood sugar monitoring remains infrequent, as in Stage 2. This is in part because these medicines do not usually cause hypoglycemia unless they are combined with insulin or sulfonylureas.

- **Sulfonylureas:**
  Another medicine choice is a sulfonylurea. These medications include DiaBeta®, Micronase®, Glynase™, Glucotrol®, Glucotrol XL®, and Amaryl®. Sulfonylureas are marketed under different brand names in other countries. There are also combination medications with both metformin and a sulfonylurea (e.g., Glucovance®). All sulfonylureas increase the person's own insulin secretion which helps regulate blood sugar levels. However, they also put the person at increased risk for hypoglycemia from their own pancreas. This means more frequent blood sugar monitoring is necessary than with other medications. The usual frequency recommended is one or two blood sugar checks per day, including one fasting value and one value one or two hours after meals. After medication levels are stable for some time, providers may suggest that blood sugar levels only be done four times/day for three days per month. The choice of this medication is due to the long term safety data, its effectiveness in lowering HbA1c values, and its relatively low cost.

- **Other medications:**
  Some healthcare-providers also prescribe medications including thiazolidinediones (mainly pioglitazone, if not in heart failure), alpha-glucosidase inhibitors (e.g., Acarbose®, Miglitol®, Voglibose®) meglitinides (e.g., Regaglinide®, Nateglinide®), bile acid sequesterants (e.g., Colesevelam®) or SGLT2 inhibitors (e.g., Invokana). These are not as commonly used at our Center.

TABLE 1

Examples of Type 2 Diabetes Medications

Name	How to take	Action	Main Side Effects
Biguinide			
metformin (Glucophage®; Glucophage XR® or metformin XR®)	Oral, 2-3 doses daily XR (long acting) once daily	Reduces liver secretion of glucose May help reduce weight	Stomach upset, diarrhea, nausea, bloating; acidosis with illness (rare)
DPP4-Inhibitors			
sitagliptin (Januvia)	Oral, once daily	Prevents GLP-1 breakdown	Stuffy or runny nose, sore throat, headache, diarrhea, stomach or back pain, nausea, hypersensitivity, pancreatitis
saxagliptin (Onglyza)	Oral, once daily	Increases glucose dependent insulin secretion	
linagliptin (Trajenta)	Oral, once daily		
vildagliptin (Galvus)	Oral, 1-2 daily	Decreases glucagon after meals	
alogliptin (Nesina)	Oral, once daily	Delays stomach emptying	
GLP-1 Analogs (also called GLP-1 receptor agonists)			
exenatide (Byetta)	Injection, 1-2 doses daily	Increases glucose dependent insulin secretion	Nausea, hypoglycemia, diarrhea, dizziness, headache
exenatide extended release (Bydureon)	Injection, once weekly	Decreases glucagon levels after meals	
liraglutide (Victoza)	Injection, once daily	Delays stomach emptying	Headache, nausea, diarrhea, and anti-liraglutide antibody formation
lixisenatide (Lyxuma)		Decreases appetite	Pancreatitis
Sulfonylureas			
glyburide (DiaBeta, Micronase, Glynase)	Oral, 1-2 doses daily	Increases insulin production from the pancreas	Low blood sugar, weight gain, bloating, nausea, heartburn, anemia
glypizide (Glocotrol, Glucatrol XL)	Oral, 1-2 doses daily XL (long acting) 1-2 doses daily		
glimepiride (Amaryl)	Oral, once daily		

- There are many other medications for type 2 diabetes that were not included on this list.
- These are the medications most commonly used at our Center.
- It is strongly recommended to read the labels and discuss your concerns with your healthcare-provider.
- All stages must include a healthy lifestyle (diet and exercise), as discussed above.
- Some of these medicines are "complex." You only need to read about the medicine you are receiving.

Most doctors caring for patients with type 2 diabetes are aware that when the HbA1c level is high (e.g., above 7.3%), the fasting sugar level must receive primary emphasis in treatment. In contrast, when the HbA1c is below this level, sugar levels after meals (post-prandial) are most important to correct. Fortunately, metformin has benefits for both situations. However, when another medicine needs to be added to metformin (HbA1c not coming down), the DPP-4 inhibitors (see above) have the greater effect on sugar levels after meals. The sulfonylureas (see above) also have some effect for people with the higher or lower HbA1c levels.*

STAGE 4: BASAL INSULIN

If oral medications do not sufficiently control blood sugar levels, insulin is often added. Most providers start with adding a basal insulin (Chapter 7), such as glargine (Lantus®), detemir (Levemir®), degludec (Tresiba®) or NPH. The previous oral medications are often continued. Some providers begin basal insulin therapy with Stage 2 (metformin). A current goal is to add basal insulin in the early stages of diabetes management and to make it simple and easy to follow. There is initial evidence that this can help preserve the person's own insulin production.

Basal insulin is usually taken at dinnertime or bedtime with an aim of reducing the morning fasting blood sugar levels. Once the fasting blood sugar level is lowered, all other blood sugar levels during the day, especially after meals and in the afternoon, are usually also lowered. When starting a basal insulin, it is important to monitor the fasting blood sugar levels. Usually, the dose of basal insulin is adjusted based on the previous one to three days of fasting blood sugar values. The starting basal insulin dose is approximately 10 units/day in the evening. However, the majority of people will eventually require about 40-45 units of basal insulin/day (0.4 to 0.6 U/Kg/day) to lower their fasting blood sugar level to approximately 110-130 mg/dL (6.1-6.7 mmol/L) and to have an acceptable HbA1c value (below 7.0 percent or 53 mmol/mol). The insulin dose is usually changed by one or two units every three to seven days based on the fasting blood sugar values. People in many Asian countries (Japan, India, and China) may require significantly lower basal insulin doses (due in part to lower BMI values). Most physicians in these countries start people with four to six units of basal insulin per day.

Whenever insulin is added as a diabetes medication, the frequency of blood sugar monitoring increases significantly. A person may check

*Monnier L, et. al. Add-on therapies to metformin in type 2 diabetes: what modulates the respective decrements in postprandial and basal glucose? Diabetes Tech & Ther; 14, 891, 2012

two to three times per day (including a fasting check) until optimal dosages are reached. Many people also check their blood sugar level in the middle of the night to avoid nocturnal hypoglycemia and to help adjust the dose of basal insulin. If low blood sugars are occurring in the night, the dose may need to be decreased, or the timing of taking the basal insulin changed. Some people do better taking it in the morning or at lunch rather than at dinner or bedtime. After blood sugar levels have reached the desired ranges, it may not be necessary to check blood sugar levels as frequently. This can be discussed with the diabetes healthcare-provider. It is important to keep in mind that the addition of insulin usually results in a small weight gain. Thus, a healthy lifestyle is equally important for this choice of treatment.

It is a common, but incorrect, belief that the addition of insulin means the last stage of the disease, or that it will result in complications of diabetes (like kidney dialysis or blindness). However, in reality, **it is the delay of starting insulin treatment that may have already resulted in the long term oomplications uf dlabetes**. When the HbA1c and blood sugar levels are very high, it is recommended to gradually bring the HbA1c level down to a target range (below 7 percent or 53 mmol/mol). Rarely, if the HbA1c level is brought down too quickly, it may result in early deterioration of eye and kidney disease. However, this deterioration usually resolves over several months and, over time, improvements in eye, kidney and nerve damage will be observed.

STAGE 5: COMBINATION OF BASAL INSULIN AND GLP-1 ANALOGS

When either basal insulin or GLP-1 analog treatment alone is not able to control blood sugar levels and the HbA1c levels continue to be above seven percent, a combination of the two can be tried. The GLP-1 analog injection is given in the morning before breakfast to lower the post-meal rise in blood sugar levels. The basal insulin is injected at bedtime to effectively lower fasting blood sugar levels. This combination, sometimes along with oral medications, is often effective in achieving the desired glucose control with minimal or no weight gain. This is due to the fact that basal insulin troatment usually results In a slight weight gain, which is neutralized by GLP-1 analog treatment.

STAGE 6: RAPID-ACTING PRE-MEAL INSULIN (along with basal insulin)

The last step in effective diabetes management for people with type 2 diabetes includes adding meal-time insulin such as aspart (NovoLog®), lispro (Humalog®), or glulisine (Apidra®), (see Chapter 7) to lower the post-meal rise in blood sugar values. In this stage of type 2 diabetes, the pancreas is not able to cope with the day-to-day needs for insulin, just as in type 1 diabetes. Most people monitor their blood sugar levels three to four times a day. This is usually done fasting in the morning, and before, or two hours after meals (to self-adjust insulin dosages of basal and meal-time insulins). The aim of checking blood sugar levels is to adjust the insulin dose so that hypoglycemia can be minimized while effectively lowering high blood sugar levels (hyperglycemia). The aim is to have all post-meal blood sugar levels below 180 mg/dL (10 mmol/L). Our experience shows that rapid-acting insulin works best if taken 15-20 minutes before meals, based on expected food content and blood sugar values. If the blood sugar value is below 90 mg/dL (5 mmol/L), it is wise to take the insulin with the meal. With this treatment regimen, usually modest weight gain occurs so that a healthy lifestyle is highly recommended.

2012 POSITION STATEMENT

A summary of the joint US/European Position Statement on the treatment of type 2 diabetes is provided in Table 2. The recommendations for management are very similar to the recommendations presented in this chapter.

SUMMARY

Management of type 2 diabetes starts with nutritional and exercise management (Stage 1). Treatment progresses to oral medications (starting in Stage 2 with metformin), and eventually leads to insulin. It is VERY important to INDIVIDUALIZE the treatment. Consulting a physician on a regular basis is important to allow NECESSARY and TIMELY changes in medications to maintain target blood sugar control. The frequency of blood sugar monitoring varies with the risk of hypoglycemia as well as the need to improve glycemic (sugar) control. Effective management has been shown to delay and/or prevent the long term complications of diabetes.

TABLE 2

US/European Position Statement on the Treatment of Type 2 Diabetes

A 2012 Position Statement on the treatment of type 2 diabetes emphasizes that patients need to be involved in decision making related to their treatment. The Position Statement, referenced below,* will be helpful to diabetes care-providers wanting more in-depth information, particularly pertaining to medications.

The Statement noted that factors to be considered in choosing a target for glycemic (sugar) control (HbA1c level) might include:

- the patient's quality of life
- the patient's attitude toward therapy
- age
- disease duration
- life expectancy
- support system
- socio-economics

Thus, a lower HbA1c level might be aimed for in a younger, healthier, motivated patient (who would be expected to live longer). The goal might be for an HbA1c level below 7.0 or 6.5 percent (53 or 48 mmol/mol). In contrast, an older patient, especially with other health problems (e.g., coronary artery disease), and/or with a greater risk of hypoglycemia, might have a higher target HbA1c level. This might be below 7.5 or 8.0 percent (58 or 64 mmol/mol).

The Position Statement agreed that lifestyle modifications should be tried first. Then, if goals are not met after three to six months, medicines such as metformin should be tried. If goals are still not met after another three to six months, other medicines such as a sulfonylurea, a thiazolidinedione (TZD) (mainly pioglitazone, if not in heart failure), a DPP-IV inhibitor, a GLP-1 analog, or basal insulin should be considered.

The Position Statement noted that because patients with type 2 diabetes are at increased risk of cardiovascular morbidity and mortality, the aggressive management of cardiovascular risk factors (blood pressure and lipid therapy, antiplatelet treatment and smoking cessation) are also important. People with kidney or liver disease also need special considerations. These recommendations are similar to the treatment approach used in our Center.

*Position Statement: Inzucchi, SE, Bergenstal, RM, Buse, JO et. al. Management of Hyperglycemia in Type 2 Diabetes: A Patient-Centered Approach American Diabetes Association. Diabetes Care 35, 1364, 2012 and European Association for the Study of Diabetes. Diabetologia 55, 1577, 2012

Don't forget to take your medication!

42

INSULIN TYPES AND ACTIVITY

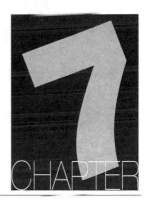

AAll people receiving insulin should know the name, type, and action time for the insulin(s) they use. Insulin is most commonly available as U-100 insulin. This means there are 100 units of insulin per cc (mL). Insulin vials usually contain 10 cc (mL) or 1,000 units of insulin. Insulin vials not currently being used must be stored so that they do not freeze or get heated over 90° F (32° C); otherwise they will spoil. The insulin vial(s) currently being used can be kept at room temperature for 30 days. Commonly used insulins and their action profiles are shown in Table 1 and Figures 1 and 2.

WHY ARE INSULIN INJECTIONS NEEDED?

- Not enough insulin is made in the pancreas of a person with type 1 diabetes. This is also sometimes true for people with type 2 diabetes, especially after the diabetes has been present for a longer time period.

- Insulin can't be taken as a pill because it would be destroyed by stomach enzymes.

- People with type 2 diabetes who initially have ketones or very high blood sugar levels usually also take insulin injections, at least in the beginning.

THE FOUR TYPES OF INSULIN (based on duration of action)

1) *"Short-acting"* (Humalog [insulin lispro], NovoLog [insulin aspart] and Apidra [insulin glulisine]) and *Regular insulin*

- Humalog, NovoLog and Apidra are also referred as **"rapid-acting"** insulins. They are more rapid-acting than Regular insulin. Their peak action is earlier and they do not last as long in the body as does Regular insulin (see Table 1).

- Humalog, NovoLog, Apidra and Regular insulins are a clear solution. They are available in vials, and are also available in insulin pens (see Chapter 8).

- Regular insulin is longer-lasting than Humalog, NovoLog and Apidra (Table 1).

- People who use an insulin pump (see Chapter 22) use only a rapid-acting insulin in the pump.

2) *"Intermediate-acting"* (NPH)

- NPH insulin is a cloudy solution and must be mixed before being drawn up into a syringe to get a consistent dose with each shot.

- The bottles should be turned gently up and down 20 times before drawing the insulin into the syringe.

- NPH insulin peaks 3-8 hours after being given and is usually taken twice daily (Figure 1 and Table 1).

- NPH insulin is commercially available pre-mixed with varying amounts of rapid-acting or Regular insulin. These combinations are available in vials and are also available in insulin pens. A 70/30 mixture indicates 70 percent NPH insulin and 30 percent rapid-acting or Regular insulin. A 50/50 mixture indicates equal amounts of both NPH and rapid-acting or Regular insulin. In Europe, a 30/70 mixture means 30 percent of Regular or short-acting insulin and 70 percent of NPH insulin. Other combinations of short-acting insulin and NPH insulin are also available.

3) *"Long-lasting"* (Lantus [insulin glargine] and Levemir [insulin detemir])

- These are basal (flat-acting with minimal peak) insulins that last approximately 24 hours (see Table 1 and Figure 2).

- They are clear insulins (don't confuse with the rapid-acting insulins).

- Both Lantus and Levemir are available in vials, and are also available in pens.

4) *"Ultra-long-lasting"* (Tresiba [insulin degludec])

A new insulin, Tresiba, has recently been approved in Europe, Japan and Mexico, but not in the U.S. Although used on a daily basis, it lasts for up to three days (72 hours). It has lower day-to-day variability of action and may reduce nighttime low blood sugars.

An ultra long-lasting insulin combined with a rapid (short)-acting insulin ("Degludec-Plus" or Ryzodeg®) is also available in Europe, Japan and Mexico, but not in the U.S. It is a commercially available pre-mixed insulin (like the 70/30 pre-mixed insulin above). This is the only ultra-long acting insulin that is pre-mixed with a rapid-acting insulin (insulin aspart). This can be started as one injection at dinnertime or before any other major meal of the day. This mixture is then effective in lowering the blood sugar levels after that meal. Less basal/ultra-long acting insulin is then needed when the combination insulin is used. Studies have shown that the total insulin dose needed may be up to 23 percent lower when compared with Lantus alone.

TABLE 1

Commonly Used Insulins

TYPE OF INSULIN*	Begins Working	Main Effect	All Gone
SHORT (RAPID)-ACTING			
Humalog/NovoLog/Apidra	15 minutes	90 minutes	3-4 hours
Regular	30-60 minutes	2-4 hours	6-9 hours
INTERMEDIATE-ACTING			
NPH	1-2 hours	3-8 hours	12-15 hours
LONG-LASTING			
Lantus (insulin glargine)	1-2 hours	2-22 hours	24 hours
Levemir (insulin detemir)	1-2 hours	2-20 hours	20-24 hours
ULTRA-LONG-LASTING			
Tresiba (insulin degludec)	1-2 hours	24 hours	72 hours

*Based on duration of activity

FIGURE 1

Example of Two Injections Per Day

HL = Humalog, NL = NovoLog, AP = Apidra, R = Regular insulin

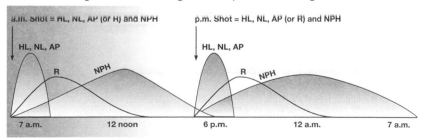

HOW AND WHEN IS INSULIN USED?

Most people with type 1 diabetes take three or more injections of insulin each day or use an insulin pump (Chapter 22). The most common insulin therapy currently used, especially for people with type 1 diabetes, is called **"Basal-Bolus Insulin Therapy."** It consists of a long-lasting or ultra-long-lasting **(basal)** insulin combined with a rapid-acting **(bolus)** insulin given prior to meals (Figure 2). The rapid-acting insulin is also used for correction of high blood sugar levels (Chapter 11). Use of the different types of insulin is discussed below.

FIGURE 2

Use of Lantus, Levemir or Tresiba Insulin with Basal-Bolus Insulin Therapy

HL = Humalog, NL = NovoLog, AP = Apidra, R = Regular insulin

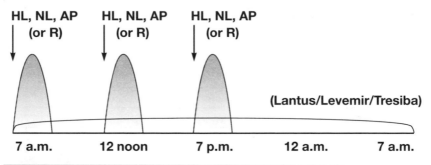

Lantus, Levemir, or Tresiba insulin are used as the basal insulin (given in the morning, or at dinner or at bedtime). A rapid-acting insulin (HL = Humalog; NL = NovoLog; AP = Apidra) is then taken 15-20 minutes prior to meals and snacks. Many people with type 2 diabetes initially take a basal insulin (Lantus, Levemir or Tresiba) once daily. The time of day can vary, but should remain consistent.

USE OF SHORT-ACTING (ALSO REFERRED TO AS RAPID-ACTING) INSULIN (HUMALOG, NOVOLOG OR APIDRA) and REGULAR INSULIN

- Rapid-acting insulin (Humalog, NovoLog or Apidra) should be taken 15-20 minutes before the meal unless the blood sugar is below 100 mg/dL (5.5 mmol/L) or is falling rapidly. If this is the case, the insulin can be given at the time of the meal (see Figure 3, Chapter 8).

- If Regular insulin is being used, the injection should be given 30-60 minutes before meals.

- Rapid-acting insulins are also used to "correct" a blood sugar level that is too high (see Correction Insulin Dose in Chapter 11).

USE OF INTERMEDIATE-ACTING INSULIN (NPH)

NPH insulin has its main effect in three to eight hours and lasts 12 to 15 hours (see Table 1). It is usually taken twice daily in a syringe mixed with a rapid-acting insulin (Figure 1). This is usually once in the morning and once in the evening. Some physicians suggest taking NPH injections 3-4 times per day. Most patients are able to mix NPH with rapid or short acting insulin in the same syringe to avoid more injections per day.

NPH insulin taken at dinner or bedtime has a peak during the night so that low blood sugars are more common compared to when a basal (long-lasting) insulin is used.

If NPH is used at bedtime (in contrast to dinnertime), it will be more apt to last through the night without causing low blood sugar.

USE OF LONG-LASTING INSULIN (LANTUS, LEVEMIR OR TRESIBA)

Most people with type 2 diabetes who begin insulin treatment initially receive one daily injection of a "basal" insulin.

It works as a "basal" insulin, which prevents the liver from producing sugar and ketones and releasing them into the blood.

The dose is usually taken without any other insulin in the syringe (or ask your doctor if it is okay to combine). If using basal-bolus therapy, then Humalog, NovoLog or Apidra insulin is taken 15-20 minutes before each meal (see Figure 2).

It is best to take the insulin in the buttocks (seat) or to give the insulin into a pinch of fat in the stomach (to make sure the insulin is going into the fat). If the insulin is accidentally given into muscle, it has greater peak activity and does not last as long. Most injection needles are short, so that injections into muscle happen primarily with thin individuals.

The long-lasting insulin action is relatively flat and the chance for a low blood sugar is reduced (particularly during the night when the basal insulin is taken in the morning).

The dose is adjusted on the basis of the morning blood sugar no matter when it is taken.

The shot can be taken in the morning, or at lunch, dinner or bedtime. All of these times work, although it is best to give it at the same time each day. If the blood sugar is consistently above the desired range at breakfast (Chapter 9), the dose should be increased. If blood sugar levels are below the desired level at breakfast, the dose should be decreased.

SUMMARY

Insulin is taken by people with diabetes to replace the insulin no longer made in adequate quantity by their own pancreas. There are several different types of insulins which vary in their time to peak action, as well as in the duration in the body. There are also different methods of taking insulin, such as through a syringe or with an insulin pen (Chapter 8). It is important to talk with your doctor about the best type of insulin, the best method of delivering it, and about making any adjustments to the dose. Insulin is a "life-saving" medicine but is not a "cure."

INSULIN PENS, DRAWING UP INSULIN FROM VIALS & INSULIN INJECTIONS

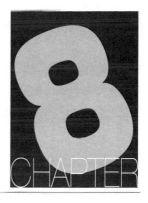

CHAPTER 8

The nurse educator or provider will teach the best way to draw up and take insulin. The first task is to draw the insulin into the syringe, or to get the insulin pen ready for use.

USE OF INSULIN PENS

Insulin pens provide convenience and accuracy. Most types of insulin are now available in pens. Using a pen is quite easy and is summarized below.

- Remove the paper tab from the needle and screw it on the end of the pen.

- Clean the skin where the shot will be given. Rotate sites daily.

- Remove the needle cover.

- Enter 2 to 3 units (by rotating the dial) in the pen as a "priming dose" and with the needle pointed upward into the air, observe that the insulin comes out.

- Dial in the number of units to be given.

- Insert the needle under the skin.

- Inject the insulin slowly. Then count 10 seconds before removing the needle. (This prevents insulin from leaking out.)

- Rub the injection site gently to close the track of the needle.

- Put the cover back on the needle. (Some say to change the needle with each injection and others say once daily.)

DRAWING UP INSULIN FROM VIALS

Prepare everything you will need, such as:

- bottles of insulin you will use

- syringe and needle

- alcohol wipe for tops of bottles

DRAWING UP ONE INSULIN INTO A SYRINGE

- Know what dose of insulin you need to take.

- Wipe off the top of the insulin bottle with an alcohol swab.

- If injecting NPH (cloudy looking insulin), gently turn the bottle up and down 20 times. This mixes the insulin so it will have a consistent strength.

- Inject air (same number of units as the insulin to be withdrawn) into the insulin bottle and leave the needle (attached to the syringe) in the bottle.*(See footnote at the bottom of next page.)

- Turn the bottle with the needle in it upside down and get rid of any air bubbles in the syringe by drawing insulin into the syringe and then slowly pushing it back into the vial until no bubbles can be seen.

- Draw up the insulin dose you need and remove the needle from the bottle.

- If the insulin bottles have been in the refrigerator, you can warm up the insulin in the syringe by holding the syringe in the closed palm of your hand for a minute. It will be less likely to sting if the insulin is at room temperature.

DRAWING UP TWO INSULINS INTO A SYRINGE

- World-wide, this often involves a mixture of NPH and Regular insulin. Some physicians use commercially pre-mixed insulin (see Chapter 7). Using pre-mixed insulin gives less flexibility for people who want to vary their dose of rapid-acting insulin (for food, exercise, etc.). However, it prevents having to draw-up two insulins in one syringe or to do two separate injections at the same time.

- Know how much of each insulin you need to give.

- Wipe off the tops of the insulin bottles with an alcohol swab.

- Inject air (same units as the insulin to be withdrawn) into the intermediate-acting (cloudy) insulin bottle with the bottle sitting upright on the table and remove the needle.*

- Inject air (same units as the insulin to be withdrawn) into the clear (rapid-acting) insulin bottle and leave the needle in the bottle.

- Turn the rapid-acting bottle with the needle in it upside down to get rid of any air bubbles in the syringe. This is done by drawing insulin into the syringe and then gently pushing it back into the bottle.

- Draw up the clear rapid-acting insulin you need and remove the needle from the bottle.

- Mix the cloudy (NPH) insulin by gently turning the bottle up and down 20 times. This mixes the insulin so that it will have a consistent strength.

- Turn the bottle upside down to put the needle into the bottle. Draw up the cloudy insulin into the syringe. **Make sure not to push any rapid-acting insulin already in the syringe back into this NPH bottle.**

- If the insulin bottles have been in the refrigerator, you can warm up the insulin once it is mixed in the syringe by holding the syringe in the closed palm of your hand for a minute. It will be less likely to sting if the insulin is at room temperature.

GIVING THE INSULIN (See Figure 1)

- Choose the area of the body where you are going to give the shot. Use two or more areas and use different sites within the area.

- Always use a different site, not the same one used in the previous injection. Examples of sites are shown in Figure 2.

- Make sure the area where you will be giving the shot is clean.

- Relax the chosen area.

*An option now used by some people is to not put air into the insulin bottles, but to just "vent" the bottles once a week to remove any vacuum. This is done by removing the plunger from the syringe and inserting the needle into the upright insulin bottle. Air will be sucked in through the needle removing the vacuum from the bottle. (The vacuum may otherwise pull insulin from the syringe back into the insulin bottle. This is most important if two insulins are being mixed in the same syringe.)

- Pull up the skin with the finger and thumb (even with short needles).

- Touch the needle to the skin and poke it through the skin as below.

For Short Needle:
- Use a 90° angle for the 5/16 inch (short) or the Ultra-Fine Nano needle. These hurt less and are not as likely to go into muscle.
- A 90° angle is straight: __↓__.

For Long Needle:
- Use a 45° angle for the 5/8 inch needle (only).
- A 45° angle looks like this: __↙__.

- Push the insulin in slowly and wait 10 seconds to let the insulin absorb.

- Let go of the pulled up skin.

- Put a finger or dry cotton over the injection site as the needle is pulled out. Gently rub a few times to close the hole where the needle was inserted. Press your finger or the cotton down on the area where you gave the shot if bruising or bleeding occurs.

LIPOATROPHY and LIPOHYPERTROPHY

When insulin is injected into the same site repeatedly, it may result in fat cells multiplying (lipohypertrophy or swelling). This may result in unreliable insulin absorption (although it can be a less painful injection site). Injection sites must be rotated.

Rarely, insulin injection sites lose fat cells with skin "denting," also called "lipoatrophy." This is usually due to the formation of insulin antibodies. Insulin absorption at these sites is not reliable. Possible solutions to this problem are suggested below.

- Change injection sites and rotate daily (see Figure 2).

- Discuss changing insulin with the physician: e.g., if taking Humalog, try NovoLog or Apidra. Similarly, try a different long-lasting insulin.

- Give insulin injections (using the new insulin) around these pits (lipoatrophy sites). This may regenerate fat cells.

- Avoiding these sites completely and changing insulin types may resolve the pits over time.

FIGURE 1

Injecting the Insulin

A. Wash hands

B. Warm and mix insulin

C. Wipe top of insulin bottle with alcohol

D. Pull out dose of insulin

E. Clean injection site

F. Pinch up skin and fat tissue

G. Inject insulin at 45° (5/8 inch) or at 90° (short or Nano needles)

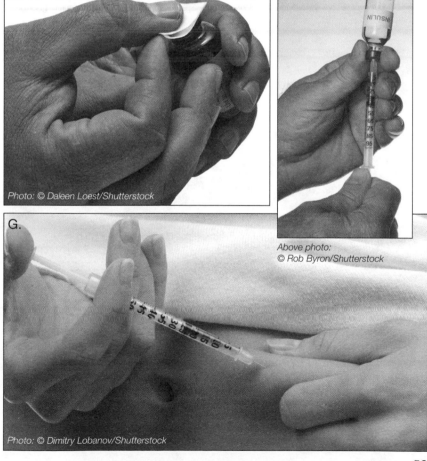

C.

Photo: © Daleen Loest/Shutterstock

D.

INSULIN

Above photo:
© Rob Byron/Shutterstock

G.

Photo: © Dimitry Lobanov/Shutterstock

WHEN TO INJECT THE INSULIN (Figure 3)

When possible, the rapid-acting insulin should be given 15 to 20 minutes prior to the meal (as discussed in Chapter 7). This will result in lower blood sugar levels after meals. Blood sugar levels from food will peak in 60 minutes (depending on contents of the food ingested) whereas the Humalog, NovoLog or Apidra will peak in 90 minutes. Absorption of insulin is usually more rapid from the abdomen and arm than from the buttocks or thigh. Regular insulin peaks in 2 hours. The effect of giving the insulin 20 minutes prior to the meal ("PRE") is shown in Figure 3. This should only be done if the blood sugar is above 90 mg/dL (5 mmol/L) and is not trending rapidly downward.

STINGING AT INSULIN INJECTION SITES

- Most of the time this is due to a difference in temperature of the insulin due to taking it out of the refrigerator.

- All pens and vials in use may be kept at room temperature to avoid stinging.

- When using a fresh pen or vial from the refrigerator, roll in between warm hands for one to three minutes to bring the temperature up to room temperature.

- Rarely, stinging may be due to an allergy associated with a specific type of insulin. In that case, ask the provider to prescribe a different insulin.

- Very rarely, some insulins (e.g., Lantus) may sting more than others due to differences in the pH (acidity). This difference in pH is more noticeable when the insulin dose is large. Again, changing to a different insulin may help.

- Higher units (volume) injected may result in stinging for any insulin. The best way to avoid this is to split the insulin dose (e.g., morning and dinnertime).

SUMMARY

Insulin is administered using an insulin pen or using a syringe with insulin drawn from a vial. The diabetes educator will teach the best method for giving insulin injections.

FIGURE 2

Injection Rotation Chart

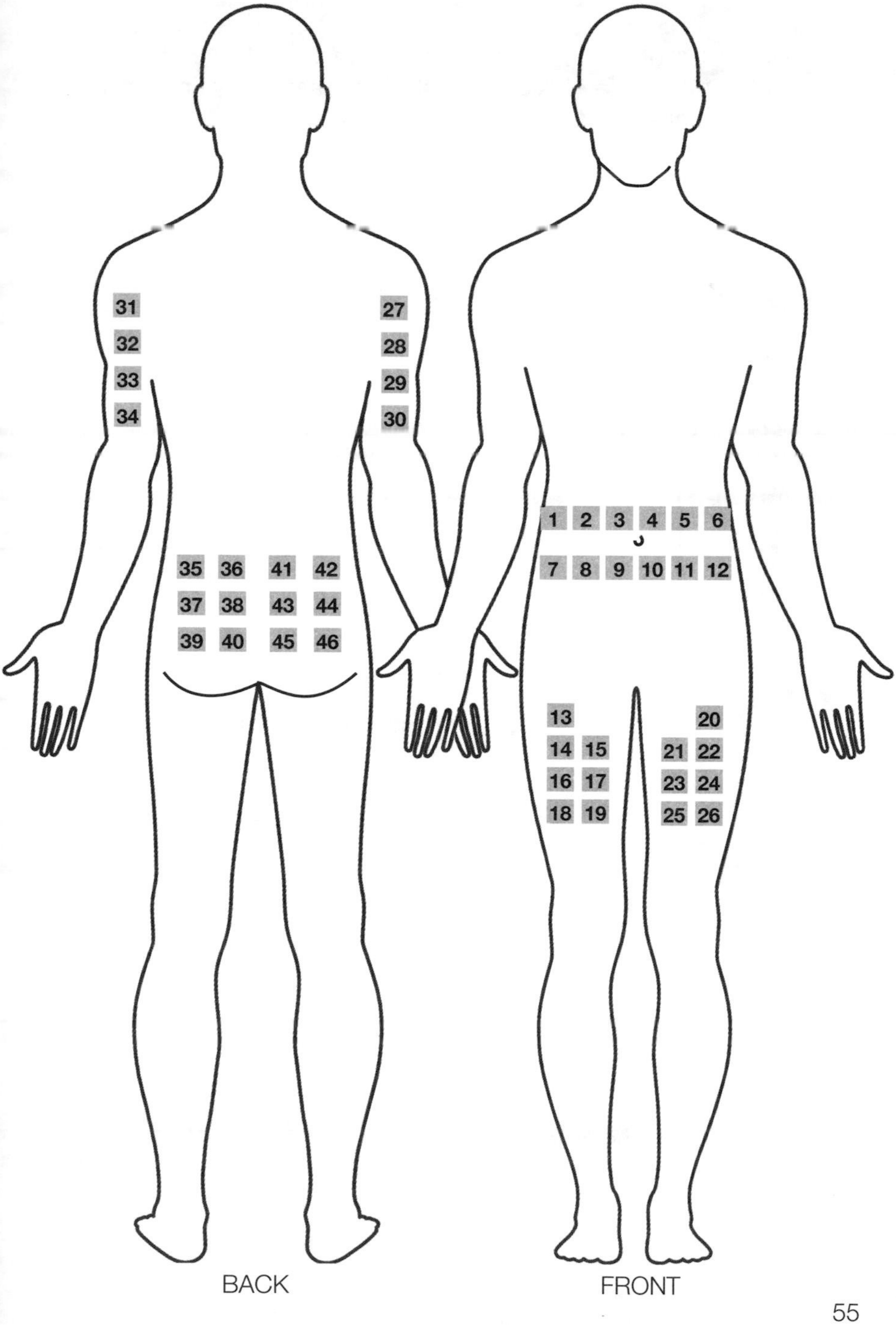

BACK   FRONT

FIGURE 3

Blood Sugar Levels Before or After a Meal

Blood sugar levels when insulin was given 20 minutes prior to a meal ("PRE"), at the beginning of the meal ("START"), or after the meal ("POST"). The ADA goal for blood sugars at any time after a meal is to not exceed 180 mg/dL (10 mmol/L).

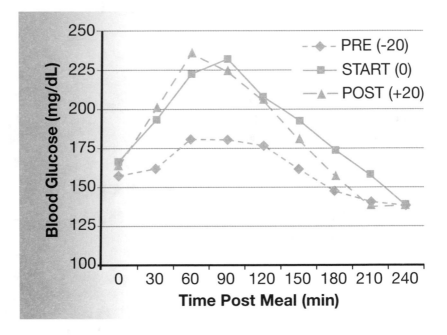

Data compliments of: Cobry E et. al. Diabetes Technology and Therapeutics 12:173, 2010

BLOOD SUGAR CHECKING

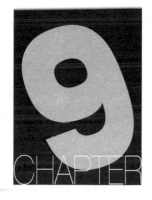

All people with diabetes (type 1 or type 2) need to know how to check blood sugar (glucose) levels. Blood sugars are measured more frequently in people with type 1 diabetes compared to people with type 2 diabetes. People with type 1 diabetes usually check their blood sugar levels at least four times a day.

People with type 2 diabetes use a variable frequency of blood sugar checking (as discussed in Chapter 6). This is often related to the stage and type of treatment. Some people just check the morning fasting blood sugar level (no food consumed for 8-10 hours). If the HbA1c level is in an optimal range (below 7.0 percent or 53 mmol/mol), this may be done once or twice weekly. If the HbA1c value is higher, blood sugar levels should be checked more frequently. Other healthcare-providers ask for several checks each day in the two weeks prior to a clinic visit. All people with diabetes having symptoms of a low blood sugar should check their blood sugar level. Whenever insulin is used, the frequency of blood sugar monitoring is greater. When adjusting the insulin dose, blood sugar monitoring should be more frequent. You should discuss the goal for the frequency of blood sugar checks with your diabetes healthcare-provider.

GOALS

The American Diabetes Association recommends that fasting and pre-meal blood sugar levels should be maintained at or below **130 mg/dL or 7.2 mmol/L**. It is recommended that blood sugar levels not exceed **180 mg/dL or 10 mmol/L** at any time after meals. Suggested target levels to aim for are shown in Table 1. You should discuss your goal for blood sugar ranges with your diabetes healthcare-provider.

HOW TO CHECK BLOOD SUGAR

Blood sugar checking involves obtaining a small sample of blood using a lancing device ("poker"). A small drop of blood is placed on a disposable test strip. A meter is then used to calculate the amount of sugar in the blood sample. The blood sample is usually taken from a fingertip. Some people use an "alternate site," such as the forearm (see below).

FINGERSTICK CHECKING

There are now many lancing devices which are used to draw the small drop of blood for sugar checking. They usually consist of a spring loaded lancet that can be set to different depths depending on skin thickness. Diabetes educators can demonstrate proper techniques for poking fingers. Some suggestions are outlined below.

- Insert the lancet into the poker, per manufacturer instruction.

- Always wash your hands with soap and warm water and make sure to dry them completely. If unable to wash hands, use an alcohol wipe and allow it to dry. **Sugar on the finger tip is a common reason for a blood sugar level to read high when the value is actually fine.**

- Poke the side or tip (not the ball) of the chosen finger by holding the lancing device against the finger and pushing the release button.

- To get enough blood, hold your hand down (below heart level) and "milk" the finger by squeezing gently from the palm to the tip of the finger.

- Put the drop of blood on the blood sugar strip as taught for each meter.

- Hold a cotton ball on the poked site to stop the bleeding.

ALTERNATE SITE CHECKING

Some meters now require such a small drop of blood that it can be obtained from the arm or another site. Each lancing device and/ or meter has specific instructions about how to obtain an alternate site blood sample. It is important to know that blood sugar values from alternate sites may lag behind the true blood sugar level from fingertips, since blood circulation may not be as good at the alternate site. Therefore, if low blood sugar levels are suspected, the fingertip must be used for the blood sugar check.

TABLE 1

	Blood/CGM Glucose Level		Possible Symptoms
	mg/dL	mmol/L	
VERY HIGH	400-800	(22.2-44.4)	Upset stomach Difficulty breathing Remember to check ketones!
HIGH	150-400	(11.1-22.2)	Low energy
GOAL Fasting and pre-meal Post meal	below 130 below 180	below 7.2 below 10	No symptoms
LOW	below 70	(below 3.9)	Sweating Hunger Shakiness
"TRUE LOW"	below 60	(below 3.3)	As with "low" above If not treated, may progress to seizure or unconscious episode
NON-DIABETIC NORMAL VALUES*			
Normal (fasting)* Normal (random)*	70-100 70-140	(3.9-5.5) (3.9-7.8)	

Most values for non-diabetic people are in this range. However, occasionally values down to 60 mg/dL (3.3 mmol/L) are still normal.

ALWAYS BRING YOUR METER AND LOG BOOK TO YOUR CLINIC VISITS!

METERS

Blood sugar meters are devices that display the blood sugar value on a screen. There is a small port for a test strip to be inserted. The steps below explain how to use a blood sugar meter.

- Remove a test strip from the vial or canister of strips.
- Insert the test strip into the strip port on the blood sugar meter.
- Some meters will require a calibration code to be set in the meter

for each new vial of strips. (Refer to owner's manual to know if this is necessary.)

- Place the blood sample on the exposed end of the test strip.
- Wait 5-10 seconds for the meter to report the blood sugar level.

There are dozens of blood sugar meters on the market today. They can be bought at pharmacies or provided by diabetes healthcare-providers. We do not recommend one meter over another. However, the meter should meet the following requirements:

- be able to store at least the last 100 values in the memory
- be able to be downloaded by the family at home and in the clinic
- require small amounts of blood to make it easier to check often

It is important to always bring the blood sugar meter to diabetes clinic appointments. The healthcare-provider can then download it and view the blood sugar values.

LOG BOOKS *(See forms at the back of this chapter.)*

Most people record blood sugar results or download meter information at regular intervals. You need to review the results to find patterns of high or low blood sugar readings on a regular (at least weekly) basis.

INTERPRETING BLOOD SUGAR LEVELS

As shown in Table 1, target blood sugar levels vary for different times of the day. Fasting and pre-meal blood sugar levels should be maintained at or below **130 mg/dL (7.2 mmol/L)**. Any values above 150 mg/dL (8.3 mmol/L) are considered elevated and may be an indication that diabetes treatment needs to be altered. Likewise, any values below 70 mg/dL (3.9 mmol/L) are considered low blood sugars, and may also require treatment changes. Post-meal blood sugar levels, ideally one or two hours after the meal, should not exceed **180 mg/dL or 10 mmol/L**. Healthcare-providers can make recommendations based on blood sugar meter downloads or logbooks. You should discuss your goals for blood sugar ranges with your diabetes healthcare-provider.

Certain chemicals may interact with blood sugar readings in some meters. Please check the directions and consult your doctor if you think this is a problem. Furthermore, if strips are expired, the blood sugar readings may also not be accurate.

It is important not to be upset about high or low blood sugar levels. This can make checking blood sugars a negative experience. It is better to simply think of the results as important information about treatment regimens. We emphasize that sugars are "in target" or "high" or "low" but never "good" or "bad." The suggestions below may help in your analysis.

- Look for patterns of highs and lows. The examples in Figure 1 of a meter download can be very helpful.

- If too many highs or lows occur, the results should be communicated to the nurse or doctor by phone, fax or email (e.g., more than two values per week above 250 mg/dL [13.9 mmol/L] or below 70 mg/dL [3.9 mmol/L]).

- We encourage patients who send blood sugar results to suggest their own solutions to their questions, which can be discussed with the doctor or nurse.

- **Always bring the meter and log book to the clinic visit. This is essential in order to obtain optimal benefit from doing blood sugar checks.** When possible, download the data prior to coming to clinic and bring it with you.

CONTINUOUS GLUCOSE MONITOR (CGM)

Diabetes management is gradually moving toward the use of a CGM. This is particularly true for people with type 1 diabetes. Use of a CGM involves wearing a sensor inserted below the skin for six to seven days each week. The sensor measures the glucose (sugar) levels in the tissue just below the skin and displays the levels on a receiver. This measurement is usually similar to the blood sugar level, but is sometimes different if the sensor is not working correctly, or if the blood sugar levels are changing rapidly. Blood sugar checking is still necessary to confirm high or low values on the CGM, and prior to determining how much insulin to give. Blood sugar levels must also be done twice daily to calibrate the CGM so that it will be as close to accurate as possible. The CGM allows glucose trends or patterns to be evaluated rather than just individual blood sugar levels. The use of a CGM is discussed in further depth in Chapter 23.

SUMMARY

Checking blood sugar levels is important for all people with diabetes. For people with type 2 diabetes the frequency varies with the stage of therapy. This should be discussed with your healthcare-provider to determine how often and at what times the checks should be done. It is important for detecting high and low blood sugars and for attaining optimal blood sugar control. It is the only way to determine how well a treatment plan is working from one day to the next. Blood sugar values are used along with HbA1c values to see how well the diabetes is being managed. It is important to bring records and meters to clinic appointments so that the diet, oral medications and/or insulin doses can be adjusted with the help of the healthcare-provider.

FIGURE 1

Example of Helpful Meter Downloads

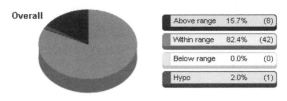

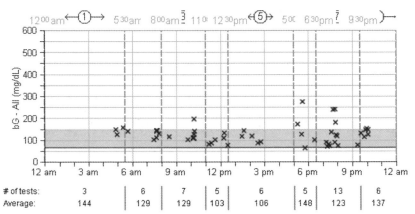

# of tests:	3	6	7	5	6	5	13	6
Average:	144	129	129	103	106	148	123	137

	12:00 am - 5:30 am	5:30 am - 8:00 am	8:00 am - 11:00 am	11:00 am - 12:30 pm	12:30 pm - 5:00 pm	5:00 pm - 6:30 pm	6:30 pm - 9:30 pm	9:30 pm - 12:00 am
Monday 04/22/2013		bG: 103 mg/dL 7:28 am						
Sunday 04/21/2013				bG: 87 mg/dL 11:24 am	bG: 87 mg/dL 2:33 pm		bG: 75 mg/dL 6:02 pm	bG: 148 mg/dL 10:04 pm
Saturday 04/20/2013				bG: 82 mg/dL 11:14 am	bG: 92 mg/dL 2:46 pm		bG: 78 mg/dL 6:21 pm	
Friday 04/19/2013		bG: 112 mg/dL 7:39 am			bG: 77 mg/dL 12:30 pm		bG: 82 mg/dL 7:24 pm	bG: 147 mg/dL 9:53 pm
Thursday 04/18/2013		bG: 131 mg/dL 7:49 am		bG: 102 mg/dL 11:38 am			bG: 71 mg/dL 7:18 pm	bG: 153 mg/dL 9:58 pm
Wednesday 04/17/2013		bG: 140 mg/dL 7:42 am		bG: 133 mg/dL 12:16 pm			bG: 91 mg/dL 7:14 pm	bG: 132 mg/dL 9:34 pm
Tuesday 04/16/2013		bG: 144 mg/dL 7:40 am		bG: 110 mg/dL 12:14 pm			bG: 74 mg/dL 7:26 pm	bG: 126 mg/dL 10:04 pm

BG Statistics

# of tests	51	Average tests/day	3.6	#of meal test pairs: 0
Average (mg/dL):	126	#HI:	0	Average meal rise: 0
SD (mg/dL):	43.6	#LO:	0	
Highest (mg/dL):	276	LBGI:	1.1	
Lowest (mg/dL):	64	HBGI:	2.5	

Examples of helpful data for your healthcare-provider to evaluate. When possible, download the data and bring it with you for your clinic visit.

LOGBOOK

PATIENT NAME: _____

Provider Return Fax: _____

Provider Return Email: _____

Provider Phone Contact: _____

Nurse Educator:_____ Physician: _____

Patient Email: _____ DOB: _____

Patient Phone: _____ Best time (8AM-5PM) to reach you?_____

Date:	Breakfast		Lunch		Dinner		Bedtime		Exercise (Time)
	Medi-cation	Dose	Medi-cation	Dose	Medi-cation	Dose	Medi-cation	Dose	Type and Duration
Sun Time:									
Mon Time:									
Tues Time:									
Wed Time:									
Thur Time:									
Fri Time:									
Sat Time:									

Current medicine and dosages:

_____

_____

_____

_____

_____

Other information (concerns, illness, weight, blood pressure, ketones, etc):

_____

_____

_____

_____

_____

Copy this page as often as you like or need

LOGBOOK

PATIENT NAME: _____

Provider Return Fax: _____

Provider Return Email: _____

Provider Phone Contact: _____

Nurse Educator: _____*Physician:* _____

Patient Email: _____ *DOB:* _____

Patient Phone: _____ *Best time (8AM-5PM) to reach you?* _____

Day/Date:

	Pre-Meal		2 hour POST Meal		Insulin Dose (if receiving)		
	mg/dl	Time	mg/dl	Time	Type	Units	Time
Breakfast							
Lunch							
Dinner							
Bedtime							

Day/Date:

	Pre-Meal		2 hour POST Meal		Insulin Dose (if receiving)		
	mg/dl	Time	mg/dl	Time	Type	Units	Time
Breakfast							
Lunch							
Dinner							
Bedtime							

Current medicine and dosages:

_____

_____

_____

_____

Other information (concerns, illness, weight, blood pressure, ketones, etc):

_____

_____

_____

_____

Copy this page as often as you like or need

LOW BLOOD SUGAR (HYPOGLYCEMIA)

CHAPTER

Hypoglycemia is defined by the American Diabetes Association (ADA) as a blood sugar level below 70 mg/dL (3.9 mmol/L). At this level, most people feel physical symptoms. When possible, a blood sugar check should be done when suspecting or feeling a low blood sugar. Low blood sugar (hypoglycemia) is uncommon for people with type 2 diabetes unless taking a sulfonylurea medicine (see Chapter 6) or insulin.

HYPOGLYCEMIA SYMPTOMS

Early symptoms include:
- hunger
- feeling shaky, sweaty and/or weak
- confusion
- sleepiness (at unusual times)/fatigue
- behavioral or mood changes
- double vision
- the signs of nighttime lows may be the same, or may include waking up alert, crying, or having bad dreams
- after a longer duration of diabetes, neurologic symptoms may occur

Later Symptoms:
- loss of consciousness
- seizure (convulsion), and then coma

A low blood sugar can come on quickly. It should be treated with approximately 15 grams of fast-acting carbohydrates either by the person (if able) or by someone who is nearby at the time. The **"rule of 15"** is to take 15 grams of rapid-acting carbohydrate (e.g., four dextrose tablets) and to recheck the blood sugar level in 15 minutes. If not treated, eventual loss of consciousness or a seizure may occur. Symptoms of different levels of hypoglycemia (mild, moderate, severe) and treatment for each level are shown in the table in this chapter.

MAIN CAUSES OF HYPOGLYCEMIA

The main causes of hypoglycemia include:

- too much insulin (or too much of an oral medication, such as a sulfonylurea)
- more exercise than usual (the low blood sugar may occur during the exercise or many hours later; Chapter 5)
- late or missed meals
- accidentally taking the wrong insulin (e.g., taking a rapid-acting insulin instead of the intended basal insulin)
- taking a bath, shower or hot tub soak too soon after an insulin injection (red, dilated skin has increased blood flow and insulin is taken up more rapidly)
- alcohol intake (see Chapter 3)

HYPOGLYCEMIA UNAWARENESS

In many subjects with long-standing diabetes, the symptoms of hypoglycemia may be absent or lost over time. This is more common in people with better sugar control. If low blood sugars are NOT being recognized by the person with diabetes, evaluation by a diabetes specialist is very important. It may be necessary to raise the target for blood sugar goals until the person is again able to recognize low blood sugar (usually in about one month). The use of continuous glucose monitoring (CGM) can also be VERY helpful in catching falling glucose levels before they result in hypoglycemia (see Chapter 23).

TREATMENT OF HYPOGLYCEMIA

The treatment of hypoglycemia is outlined in the table. If experiencing hypoglycemia, a blood sugar level should be done if possible. It is important for family members, friends and co-workers to have some knowledge of the symptoms and treatment of hypoglycemia. If the low blood sugar occurs during exercise, the person must stop exercising until the blood sugar level is back up to a normal level (ideally shown by a blood sugar check with a fingerstick).

- With **mild hypoglycemia**, 4 ounces (1/2 cup) of juice or sugared pop/soda, or 4 dextrose tablets can be taken. This is about 15g of carbohydrate and usually raises the blood sugar level in 10 to 20 minutes. If possible, the person should recheck the blood sugar level in 15-20 minutes to make sure it has come back up. If the blood sugar has not increased by then, it may be necessary to repeat the treatment. As the body gives the message to EAT, EAT, EAT, it is important to not over treat lows by eating too much and cause high blood sugars.

TABLE 1

Hypoglycemia: Treatment of Low Blood Sugar (B.S.)

Low Blood Sugar Category	MILD	MODERATE	SEVERE
Alertness Symptoms	**ALERT** • Mood changes • Shaky • Sweaty • Hungry • Fatigue • Weak • Pale	**NOT ALERT** • Lack of focus • Headache • Confused, • "Out of Control" (clumsy, etc.) • *Can't* self-treat	**UNRESPONSIVE** • Loss of consciousness • Seizure
Actions to Take	• Check B.S.** • Give 4 oz (1/2 cup) of sugary liquid. • Recheck B.S. in 10-15 min. • If B.S. <70 mg/dL (<3.9 mmol/L)*, repeat sugary fluid and recheck B.S. in 10-20 min. • If B.S. >70 mg/dL (>3.9 mmol/L), give solid snack.*	• *Place in a position of safety* • Check B.S. • Those on insulin pump, may disconnect or suspend until fully recovered from low B.S. **(awake and alert).** • Give Insta-Glucose or cake decorating gel — put between gums and cheek and rub cheek. • Look for person to 'wake-up.' Recheck B.S. in 10-20 min. • *Once alert —* follow "actions" under 'Mild' column.	• *Place in a position of safety* • Check B.S. • Those on insulin pump may disconnect or suspend until fully recovered from low B.S. **(awake and alert).** • Glucagon — best to give into muscle, 100 units (all of dose or 1cc) • If giving full 100 unit dose, may use syringe in box and inject through clothing and into thigh. • **Check B.S. every 10-15 min. until >70 mg/dL (>3.9 mmol/L).** • **If no response, may need to call 911.** • If above 70 mg/dL (3.9 mmol/L), **check B.S. every hour for 4-5 hours.** • High risk for more lows X 24 hours (need to increase food intake and decrease insulin doses).
Recovery Time	10-20 minutes	20-45 minutes	Effects can last 2-12 hours. **Call RN/MD and report the episode.**

*< means less than; *> means more than

**B.S. means blood sugar

- With **moderate hypoglycemia**, if the person is acting "confused" or "out of it," another person will need to help. Since liquids are a swallowing risk at this point, glucose gel or cake frosting can be used and placed in between the gums and cheeks. Rub the outer cheek to increase absorption of the gel. The person doing the treatment should stay with the hypoglycemic person until the blood sugar level has returned to normal. Low-dose glucagon (see below) is also sometimes given.

- With a **severe reaction**, the person may be unconscious or may have a seizure (jerking movements). Give a 1 mL (1cc) of glucagon (1 mg) by injection into the muscle as described below.

GLUCAGON

Glucagon is a synthetic form of a naturally occurring hormone also made in the islet cells of the pancreas (in the alpha cells). It has the opposite effect of insulin and raises the blood sugar levels. It does this by making the liver release sugar into the bloodstream and can raise blood sugar levels in 10 to 20 minutes.

HOW TO GIVE A GLUCAGON INJECTION

- Open the glucagon kit and take out the syringe which contains a liquid inside of it.

- Remove the needle cap and inject all of the liquid into the powder vial. Then mix the vial by turning up and down.

- After mixing, draw the entire solution into the syringe and use the large needle for injection into muscle: This could be into the outer thigh or upper/outer buttocks.

- Glucagon will make the blood sugar rise, usually in 10 to 20 minutes. If glucagon is not available, or if the person does not respond in 10 to 20 minutes, the paramedics (911) should be called.

- Though the result of giving glucagon is the opposite of giving insulin, it is NOT sugar. It is a hormone, like insulin.

- After the person is awake and able to swallow, liquids or food can be offered. Continue to check blood sugar levels. However, glucagon sometimes can cause an upset stomach (nausea or vomiting).

- Your doctor or nurse should be called before the next insulin is given. The amount of insulin you give may need to be reduced. Having a severe low blood sugar increases the likelihood of another severe low blood sugar in the next few days.

LOW-DOSE GLUCAGON

If a person has a low blood sugar and can't keep food down, or has difficulty getting the blood sugar back up, low-dose glucagon can be given under the skin (just like insulin). The dose for an adult is 15 units. Prepare the glucagon as you would for a full injection by mixing the entire vial with all of the liquid from the large syringe. However, for low-dose glucagon, it can be given using an insulin syringe with measurements to 15 units. The dose can be repeated every 20 to 30 minutes until the blood sugar level is back up. This use is different than giving the full dose for someone who is unconscious. Low-dose glucagon treatment has prevented many emergency room visits. The mixed glucagon usually forms a gel in 24 hours and must then be discarded. However, until it gels it can be reused. It is important not to forget to refill the glucagon prescription once it has been used.

IF A SEIZURE OR LOSS OF CONSCIOUSNESS OCCURS, GIVE A GLUCAGON INJECTION.

- **For most adults, give the entire vial (1 mg, 1 ml, 100 units).**
- **If no response in 10 to 20 minutes, call 911.**

DRIVING WITH DIABETES

When taking metformin, GLP-1 analogs, DPP4-inhibitors (as detailed in Chapter 6) alone, low blood sugars are not a concern. Thus, checking blood sugar levels before driving is not necessary.

However, when taking insulin (of any kind) and/or a sulfonylurea medicine, alone or in combination with other medications, low blood sugars can occur. It is then essential to check a blood sugar (or CGM) level prior to driving a car or vehicle. It has been shown that driving with a low blood sugar level results in greater impairment than when driving drunk. If you feel low while driving, it is essential to pull over and have a snack. You should never assume you can "make it" home or to the nearest convenience store. You should not resume driving until a repeat blood sugar level has returned to normal or is at least above 70 mg/dL (3.9 mmol/L). Snacks (a small can of juice, granola bar, etc.) should be kept in the car and be easily accessible.

PSYCHOLOGICAL ASPECTS

The fear of hypoglycemia is common for people with diabetes as well as for family members. This can sometimes make people afraid of having optimal control of their diabetes and taking the correct medications. Education about hypoglycemia is the best way to alleviate this fear.

SUMMARY

The person with diabetes, as well as family members and friends, must know how to recognize and treat low blood sugars. Education from a diabetes specialist is important. Glucagon must be available in an easy-to-find place and always taken along when traveling.

HIGH BLOOD SUGAR (Hyperglycemia)

CHAPTER 11

HIGH BLOOD SUGAR

High blood sugar (hyperglycemia) can be the result of many different causes, including:

- illness (see Chapter 13)
- forgetting to take insulin or other medications
- too low a dose of insulin or other medications
- eating too many carbohydrates
- stress
- physical trauma (e.g., accident, surgery, heart attack, etc.)
- for people using an insulin pump, having the infusion tubing become plugged or come out from under the skin
- "spoiled" insulin (frozen or above 90°F or 32°C)
- taking medications that increase blood sugars (e.g., steroids)

ACUTE ELEVATIONS OF BLOOD SUGAR LEVELS

High blood sugars can occur for a short period **(acute)**, or over a longer period **(chronic)**. With acute hyperglycemia (e.g., an illness), there may be a sudden onset of symptoms. These may include any of the following:

- thirst
- frequent urination
- dry mouth
- lack of energy
- blurred vision

Blood sugar monitoring will detect any acute increases in blood sugar levels. As discussed in Chapter 9, the goal is to have a fasting or pre-meal blood sugar value below 130 mg/dL or 7.2 mmol/L. The post-meal blood sugar level should be below 180 mg/dL or 10 mmol/L. Values above 250 mg/dL or 13.9 mmol/L generally require special attention and ketone checking (see Chapter 12).

For people taking insulin who have a blood sugar levels in the range of 150-250 mg/dL (3.9-13.9 mmol/L), the treatment is often with a single correction dose of insulin (see Correction Insulin Doses on the following page). Blood sugar levels above 250 mg/dL (13.9 mmol/L) require special attention, and ketone levels also need to be checked. It is important to determine **WHY** the blood sugar levels are out of range. If the blood sugar was checked shortly after eating, the rise may be due to food eaten before the insulin had a chance to work. If it was an incorrect insulin dose or if food was eaten without taking insulin, the blood sugar level may respond to extra insulin quickly. If the insulin has spoiled, or if the insulin pump catheter was pulled out or plugged, or with illness or menses, more aggressive action may be needed. If the cause of the high blood sugar is not found, the levels may continue to rise.

CHRONIC ELEVATIONS OF BLOOD SUGAR LEVELS

Chronic elevations in blood sugar levels are often detected when an HbA1c level is measured (Chapter 2). The symptoms describe above for acute elevations may or may not be present. The cause may be related to obvious factors such as:

- stopping an exercise program
- indiscriminate eating
- stress
- missing medications
- illness

Sometimes the physician must do a thorough evaluation to attempt to find the cause. Infections (e.g., yeast, skin, gums) occur more frequently when blood sugar levels have been high for long periods of time. Chronic fatigue may also be present. The standard of outpatient care is to have the HbA1c level (Chapter 2) determined every three to six months. With even mild chronically elevated blood sugar values, the sugar attaches to the red blood cell protein, hemoglobin, and transforms it into hemoglobin A1c (HbA1c). Elevated HbA1c values often indicate a need to increase the dose of a medicine, add a new medicine or, with type 2 diabetes, initiate insulin treatment. The insulin dose may need to be increased if the person is already receiving insulin. Chronic elevations of blood sugar and hemoglobin A1c levels increase the risk for the microvascular and macrovascular complications of diabetes (see Chapters 16 and 17). It is thus **VERY** important to detect and correct chronic high blood sugar levels.

CORRECTION INSULIN DOSES

People taking a rapid (short)-acting insulin (Chapter 7) should know their correction insulin dose. This is the number of units of insulin needed to correct or reduce a blood sugar to a desired level (see Table 1). When choosing a dose of rapid-acting insulin, it is important to think about both the blood sugar level and the food to be eaten. For people using a continuous glucose monitor (CGM), the trend arrows on the monitor can be very helpful in determining the dose. For example, the person may choose to take less or no insulin if the glucose levels are trending rapidly downward. The correction insulin dose can be given alone or in combination with the insulin to cover food (see Table 1).

The goal is to return the blood sugar level to the desired range. A correction dose is generally given when no Humalog/NovoLog/Apidra has been given within the previous two hours. The most common correction dose is one unit of rapid-acting insulin for each 50 mg/dL (2.8 mmol/L) of blood sugar above 100 mg/dL (5.5 mmol/L). Corrections may be adjusted to connect to a higher blood sugar level (e.g., 150 mg/dL [8.3 mmol/L]) during the night. People who are using a rapid-acting insulin should discuss their correction doses with their diabetes care-provider.

TABLE 1

Example of Insulin Adjustments

Blood Sugar		Correction Factor*	Carb Unit**	Total Units of Insulin
mg/dL	mmol/L	Units of Insulin	15g Carb per unit	
150	8.3	0	1	1
200	11.1	1	2	3
250	13.9	2	3	5
300	16.7	3	4	7
350	19.4	4	5	9

*Assuming a correction factor of one unit of rapid-acting insulin per 50 mg/dL (2.8 mmol/L) above 150 mg/dL (8.3 mmol/L).

**One Carb Unit = 15g carbohydrate in this example. One unit of insulin is then given for each 15 grams of carbohydrate (see Chapter 4).

KETONES

Checking for ketones is reviewed in Chapter 12. The first clue indicating a need to check for ketones is usually a high blood sugar. Many physicians recommend checking for ketones if the morning fasting blood sugar or any two consecutive blood sugars are above 250 mg/dL (13.9 mmol/L), or **ANYTIME** there is a value above 300 mg/dL (16.7 mmol/L).

INSULIN PUMP THERAPY

Special issues with high blood sugar levels for people using an insulin pump are discussed in Chapter 22. The most common causes of acute elevations are missing an insulin dose (bolus) for food or plugging or dislodging of the insulin infusion catheter. Chronic blood sugar elevations usually require changes in insulin dosage and/or consistency in food bolus administration.

CONTINUOUS GLUCOSE MONITORING (CGM)

One of the advantages of using a continuous glucose monitor (CGM) is to have an alarm that will warn about high (or low) glucose (sugar) levels (see Chapter 23). The percent of glucose values within the desired range almost always improves when a CGM is consistently worn. Likewise, the fluctuations in glucose levels usually improve. The improvements are related to observing the alarms as well as to observing the trends of glucose values. Proper use of CGM data through education is essential. At home, you should download the CGM data onto a computer to recognize glucose trends and make necessary adjustments. You should discuss adjustments during the visit with your diabetes care-provider.

SUMMARY

Correction of acute and chronic high blood sugar levels is important. Recognizing the cause helps to determine the most appropriate way to manage them. Chronic high blood sugar levels increase the risk for long term complications of diabetes.

KETONES, DIABETIC KETOACIDOSIS (DKA) and Hyperosmolar Hyperglycemic State (HHS)

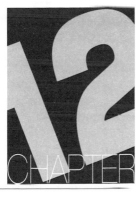

DIABETIC KETOACIDOSIS (DKA)

Ketones are formed when fat is broken down to be used for energy (Figure 1). This occurs in non-diabetic people when they fast, although usually not to high levels. Ketones occur in people with diabetes when there is not enough insulin to provide energy from carbohydrates or protein. Ketones can then build up to dangerously high levels. If this happens, a dangerous condition called diabetic ketoacidosis (DKA) can result.

HYPEROSMOLAR HYPERGLYCEMIC STATE (HHS)

Another condition, known as hyperosmolar hyperglycemic state (HHS), occurs most frequently in older people with type 2 diabetes. It is associated with dehydration, high blood sugar levels (hyperglycemia), and frequently other illnesses (Figure 1). Although HHS is less frequent than DKA in people with type 2 diabetes, it is more dangerous and may result in death in up to 20 percent of cases. It usually does not include the acidosis found with DKA. However, the two conditions can coexist together in up to 30 percent of episodes. These emergencies, DKA and HHS, are usually preventable with optimal patient compliance, adherence to care, and availability of medical care. When either HHS or DKA occurs, the precipitating cause must be found in order to prevent further episodes.

DIAGNOSIS/SYMPTOMS OF HHS AND DKA

The symptoms of **HHS** may develop slowly over days or weeks. They are often the symptoms of high blood sugar, such as:

- increased urination (polyuria)
- weight loss
- dry mouth/tongue

- weakness
- dizziness
- neurologic complaints, such as confusion

The same symptoms can occur with **DKA,** although additional symptoms/signs can include:

- labored breathing
- increased drinking (polydipsia)
- acetone (sweet) smell to the breath
- upset stomach/vomiting

These latter symptoms are due to the acidosis, which is less apt to occur with HHS.

All people with diabetes must know what ketones are, when and how to check for ketones, and what to do when ketones are found.

CAUSES OF KETONES

The main causes of ketones are:

- forgetting to give one or more insulin doses or diabetes medicines (the most common cause of DKA in patients with known diabetes)

- giving "spoiled" insulin that either got too hot (over 90°F, 32°C) or froze

- an illness causing increased insulin needs

- when not enough insulin is being taken (dose too small)

- an insulin pump that is not delivering insulin (usually due to a kinked, obstructed, or dislodged infusion catheter; see Chapter 22)

- traumatic stress on the body

HOW TO CHECK FOR KETONES

Urine Ketones

The easiest method to check for ketones is to use a urine ketone strip (e.g., Ketostix® or Chemstrip K®). After the strip is dipped into a urine sample, the color indicator will turn a shade of purple which is then compared to the color chart on the bottle. People with type 2 diabetes who have moderate or large urine ketones usually need to call their diabetes doctor or nurse for further advice. A method to check for ketones should be taken along on all trips (in case of illness or other problems).

All urine ketone test strips must be thrown out six months after the bottle has been opened. The two most common brands of urine ketone strips are:

1. Ketostix: The strip is dipped into the urine and removed immediately. After exactly 15 seconds, the strip is compared to the color chart on the vial and read as negative, trace, small, moderate, large, or extra large.

2. Chemstrip K: The strip is dipped into the urine and removed immediately. After exactly 60 seconds, the strip is compared to the color chart on the vial and read as negative, trace, small, moderate, large, or extra large.

Blood Ketones

Some people prefer to use the Precision Xtra™ meter to measure blood ketones. The steps to measure a blood ketone level are listed below.

- First, the meter must be calibrated using the purple calibration strip. This is included in every box of ketone strips.

- Next, the blood ketone strip is inserted into the meter with the three black bars facing up.

- Then, a drop of blood is applied to the white area at the end of the test strip.

- The blood ketone result (in mmol/L) will appear in 10 seconds.

Table 1 shows approximate comparisons between urine and blood ketone measurements and actions to take.

WHEN TO CHECK FOR KETONES

Ketones must be checked:

- with the signs or symptoms outlined above (under "Diagnosis/Symptoms")

- during any illness

- with a very high blood sugar level (e.g., above 300 mg/dL [16.7 mmol/L])

- if a medication is missed (especially insulin, if currently taking)

- after vomiting, even once

- with a blockage of an insulin pump catheter (if on an insulin pump)

For people who are taking insulin, if ketones are present, extra insulin may need to be given to stop the ketones from being made. **For people not taking insulin (e.g., earlier type 2 diabetes),** the diabetes healthcare-provider should be called if moderate or large urine ketones (or a blood ketone level above 1.0 mmol/L) are present. It may be necessary to give a rapid-acting insulin for a period until the cause of the increased ketone production is found and corrected.

TABLE 1
Comparison of Blood and Urine Ketone Readings

Blood Ketone	Urine Ketone		Action to take
(mmol/L)	Strip color	Level	
less than 0.6	slight/no color change	negative	normal - no action needed
0.6 to 1.0	light purple	small to moderate	extra insulin and fluids**
1.1 to 3.	dark purple	moderate to large*	call MD or RN
greater than 3.0	very dark purple	very large*	go directly to the E.R.

It is usually advised to call a healthcare-provider for a blood ketone level greater than 1.0 mmol/L or with urine ketone readings of moderate to large.

**If the blood sugar level is below 150 mg/dL (8.3 mmol/L), a liquid sugar (e.g., juice) should be taken so more insulin can be safely given.*

PREGNANCY AND KETONES

It is important to avoid DKA or ketones at all costs during pregnancy as these may result in induction of labor and/or premature delivery (see Chapter 15). During pregnancy, if blood sugar levels stay above 180 mg/dL (10 mmol/L), checking for ketones is recommended. Adjusting the insulin dose will hopefully avoid the future occurrence of ketones.

FIGURE 1

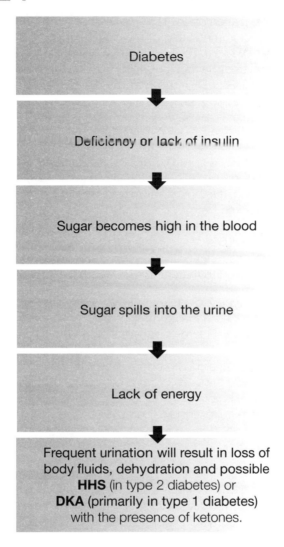

Diabetes

Deficiency or lack of insulin

Sugar becomes high in the blood

Sugar spills into the urine

Lack of energy

Frequent urination will result in loss of body fluids, dehydration and possible **HHS** (in type 2 diabetes) or **DKA** (primarily in type 1 diabetes) with the presence of ketones.

TREATMENT OF HHS OR DKA

People who have symptoms of **HHS** or **DKA** need to call their healthcare-provider immediately, or may need to go to an urgent care clinic or emergency room. DKA and HHS are serious conditions and may need special treatment in a hospital setting. It is important to find the cause of the HHS or DKA, both to reverse the illness and also to prevent it from occurring again.

People who have moderate to large ketone levels should call their diabetes healthcare-provider immediately. This condition can sometimes be treated at home by giving additional shots of a rapid-acting insulin, drinking extra liquids to help flush ketones out into the urine, and by resting. It is best to avoid exercise when having elevated ketones because exercise may cause the ketone level to increase. Finally, people taking metformin (Glucophage) should stop this medicine until the ketones have gone away. If the ketone levels are not going down with treatment or the person is showing symptoms of HHS or DKA, it is best to go to the emergency room.

Some people with type 2 diabetes who have not been receiving insulin may need to begin insulin therapy if they are found to have ketones. As noted above and in Figure 1, dehydration and **HHS** result from inadequate fluid intake. If inadequate insulin is being made to allow sugar to be used for energy, stored fat is broken down for energy. Ketones are the "side product" of fat breakdown. It is important to reverse the process before high ketone buildup occurs and **DKA** results. This often requires insulin therapy.

SUMMARY

Diabetic ketoacidosis (DKA) and hyperosmolar hyperglycemic state (HHS) can be dangerous. Patients and families must be aware of the symptoms and should know how to check for ketones. If either condition is suspected, your physician should be called; if unavailable, you may need to go to an emergency room.

SICK-DAY AND SURGERY MANAGEMENT

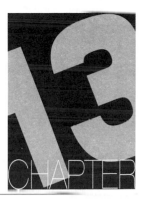

SICK-DAY MANAGEMENT

People with diabetes get sick just like other people. Any illness can affect blood sugar control. Table 1 may help you decide when to call your diabetes care-provider for help.

HIGH BLOOD SUGAR AND KETONES

General guidelines:

- Always check urine and/or blood ketones and blood sugar levels with any illness. Check ketones even if the blood sugar level is normal.

- Call your diabetes doctor or nurse if the urine ketone result is moderate or large, or if the blood ketone level is above 1.0 mmol/L.

- If you are taking metformin (Glucophage), and you have positive ketones, you may stop taking pills while you are ill. Discuss with your provider.

- People with type 2 diabetes who are not on insulin may need to receive insulin injections during an illness if blood sugar and ketone levels are high.

If you take insulin:

- Do NOT skip an insulin dose just because vomiting or other problems are present. Some insulin must still be taken, but it might need to be reduced.

- The earlier you treat elevated ketones with extra Humalog, NovoLog, Apidra or Regular insulin and with increased fluid intake, the less chance you will have of going to the hospital for diabetes care.

VOMITING

- Table 2 outlines care for vomiting when ketones are not present. If urine ketones are moderate or large, or blood ketones are above 1.0 mmol/L, the diabetes doctor or nurse should be called.

- If you take insulin and vomiting is present and ketones are negative, some insulin must still be taken. However, the insulin dose or other medicine dosages may need to be lowered. Insulin helps to keep the body from producing ketones. If the person vomits three or more times, the doctor may prescribe an orally dissolving tablet called Zofran®. Zofran suppresses vomiting. Phenergan® or Reglan® tablets or Phenergan suppositories (if vomiting prevents the ability to keep a pill down) are also sometimes helpful.

TABLE 1

Sick-Day Management:
When/Whom to Call for Emergency Care

- If you have vomited more than three times and can keep nothing in your stomach and urine ketones are not moderate or large (or blood ketones above 1.0 mmol/L), call your primary healthcare-provider.

- If help is needed with the dose of an oral medication or with an insulin dose, call your diabetes healthcare-provider.

- If moderate or large ketones are present or blood ketones are above 1.0 mmol/L, call your diabetes healthcare-provider.

- If you have difficulty breathing or have "deep breathing," you need to go to an emergency room immediately. This usually indicates severe acidosis (ketoacidosis; see Chapter 12).

- If there is any unusual behavior such as confusion, slurred speech, double vision, inability to move or talk, or jerking movements, and the blood sugar is low, someone should give sugar or instant glucose as these are signs of severe hypoglycemia. Glucagon (1.0cc [100 units]) is given if the person is unconscious or if a convulsion (seizure) occurs. In case of a convulsion or loss of consciousness, it may be necessary to call the paramedics or to go to an emergency room. Have an emergency number posted by the phone.

- Keep in mind the side effects of glucagon (e.g., nausea, vomiting).

DEHYDRATION

- Prevention of dehydration is important for illness recovery (see Table 2).

- Suggestions for sick-day fluids are giving water alternating with juice, Gatorade or sugar soda (depending on the blood sugar level).

LOW BLOOD SUGAR WITH GLUCAGON USAGE

- High blood sugar levels (± ketones) are more common with illness but low blood sugar levels are possible too. This is particularly true if the person is receiving insulin, and/or is vomiting (resulting in no food to keep the blood sugar up). If food cannot be kept down and the blood sugar is low or is falling, low-dose glucagon can be given.

- The glucagon can be mixed and given with an insulin syringe. See Chapter 11 for directions.

- The dose of glucagon is much lower (15 units) than the dose given for severe hypoglycemia (100 units [or 1cc]). If the full 100 unit dose is given, hyperglycemia (high blood sugars) may result. Also, it can worsen nausea and vomiting and formation of mild ketones.

- **Glucagon should not be given if urine ketones are moderate or large or if blood ketones are above 1.0 mmol/L. Call your doctor if this is found.**

- Call your doctor or nurse before giving the low-dose (15 units) glucagon injection if you have questions. It can be repeated every 20 minutes if needed.

- Low-dose glucagon has prevented many emergency room visits.

MEDICATIONS

Many medications (e.g., an antihistamine used for a cold) have a warning label stating that a person with diabetes should not use the medicine. This may be because it raises blood sugar levels a few points.

- If the medicine is needed, and has been discussed with a healthcare-provider previously, go ahead and take it, but watch blood sugar levels closely and correct as needed with insulin.

- Steroids (e.g., prednisone, or asthma medications) are the most difficult when trying to keep blood sugar levels in range and, if prescribed, the diabetes care-provider should be notified. If solely on oral diabetes medications, you may need to be treated with insulin for a few days. This is because steroids cause insulin resistance and a faster increase in blood sugar levels. Also, people with type 2 diabetes who are on steroids are more prone to develop hyperosmolar diabetes coma as discussed in Chapter 12.

- Pain medications (e.g., Vicodin® or Percocet®) after surgery may either raise or lower blood sugar levels. The diabetes care team will suggest ways to handle any changes in blood sugar levels.

- Some blood pressure medications (e.g., ß-blockers, calcium channel blockers, statins, and thiazide diuretics) also can cause a change in blood sugar levels and may require closer monitoring.

SURGERY MANAGEMENT

If surgery is planned, call the provider **AFTER** finding out the time of the surgery. Also find out the timing and amounts of food to be allowed post-op. Remember to notify the surgeon about diabetes and medications used.

Take diabetes supplies along with you to the surgery, such as:

- blood sugar meter and strips, with finger poker (lancet)
- insulin and syringes/pens
- oral medications
- glucose (dextrose) tablets or gel
- blood ketone strips and meter or urine ketone strips
- glucagon emergency kit
- if on an insulin pump, extra infusion sets in case they need to be changed

Take the phone card with your diabetes healthcare-provider's numbers. If you are receiving a basal insulin (Lantus, Levemir or Tresiba) or use an insulin pump, the basal insulin can be continued during the period of surgery. The dose of long-lasting basal insulin may need to be split or adjusted (call your diabetes care-provider). Then restart bolus insulin therapy when able to eat. Basal insulin may need to be increased if the surgery requires bed rest or a decrease in normal daily activity. This may also be due to the stress associated with surgery that further raises blood sugar levels.

TABLE 2

Management of Vomiting (Without Ketones)*

Avoid solid foods until the vomiting has stopped.

If vomiting is frequent, some doctors recommend giving an orally dissolving tablet called Zofran, to reduce the vomiting. It may be best to wait an hour to give fluids, until the medicine begins to work. Reglan or Phenergan (oral, topical or by rectal suppository) can also be used.

Prevent Dehydration and Low Blood Sugar

Gradually start liquids (juice, water, etc.) in small amounts. Juices (especially orange) are acceptable if the blood sugar is low. They also replace salts that are lost with vomiting or diarrhea. It is important to prevent dehydration.

- Start with a tablespoon of liquid every 10-20 minutes.

- If the blood sugar level is below 100 mg/dL (5.5 mmol/L), sugar pop or other liquids containing sugar can be given.

- If the blood sugar level is below 70 mg/dL (3.9 mmol/L) and the person is vomiting, give low-dose glucagon just as you would give insulin. The dose is 15 units. Repeat doses can be given every 20 minutes as needed.

- If the blood sugar level is above 150 mg/dL (8.3 mmol/L), do not give sugary drinks such as soda or juice.

- If there is no further vomiting, gradually increase the amount of oral fluids.

- If vomiting restarts, it may again be necessary to rest the stomach for another hour and then restart with small amounts of fluids. A repeat Zofran tablet can be given after three or four hours.

After a few hours without vomiting, gradually return to a normal diet. Soups are often helpful starters, providing needed nutrients.

*If ketones are moderate or large in the urine, or above 1.0 mmol/L in the blood, the diabetes doctor or nurse should be called.

SUMMARY

When a person with diabetes is sick, especially in the presence of vomiting or diarrhea, attention to hydration and to blood sugar and ketone levels is crucial. Low blood sugars should be promptly corrected with dextrose tablets, juice, or, if vomiting persists, an injection of glucagon. For surgery, discuss strategies with the diabetes care team.

PSYCH/SOCIAL ASPECTS OF DIABETES

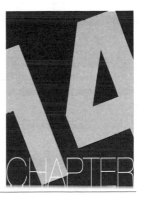

*Emily Westfall, BA, BS, H. Peter Chase, MD,
Satish K. Garg, MD*

Being diagnosed with diabetes will cause a variety of new feelings and emotions. Having these feelings is normal. It is important to discuss them and try not to let these feelings affect you negatively.

INITIAL FEELINGS

Some of the most common initial feelings are the following:

- shock
- grief
- denial
- sadness
- anger
- fear/anxiety
- guilt
- trouble adapting

As time passes, these feelings will change and life will become more normal.

It is recommended that all people speak with a counselor at diagnosis. Changes in health and daily routines can be addressed. If family members will be involved in the care and/or are affected by the diagnosis, they might also wish to speak with the counselor. All people involved need to work toward feeling positive about how diabetes will fit into their life.

Most diabetes clinics employ a social worker or counselor or are able to recommend someone who has experience with diabetes. Bring up any emotions you are having related to diabetes at your normal diabetes appointment. If a social worker or therapist is not available at your provider's office, discuss the issues further with the provider's team. Trouble coping with diabetes is common and getting help is *not* a weakness!

ADJUSTMENT

Making life with diabetes as normal as possible is the major long-term goal. Living with diabetes will gradually become easier. Adjustment continues to improve after the first few weeks and the first few months.

As time passes, the tasks below will become easier:

- exercising daily
- following healthy food choices
- adjusting medications (especially insulin) for exercise
- remembering to take medications (including insulin, if using)
- checking blood sugar levels (if asked to do so)
- counting carbohydrates (if asked to do so)
- doing other daily diabetes related tasks

Talking about diabetes at home and/or with the diabetes care team may help to reduce stress and create a comfortable schedule.

SUPPORT

If and when diabetes becomes overwhelming, talk to others who understand and can help. There are many support groups made up of people with diabetes and their family members. There are also a multitude of events that bring the diabetes community together to give strength and support to one another.

Groups of people who have diabetes may go to social events, organize conferences and arrange pot-lucks. Most of all, group activities provide a way for people with diabetes to express frustration or to exchange tips. Sometimes people might prefer to not talk about diabetes at all. Ask the diabetes healthcare-provider or look online for groups that meet in your area.

Diabetes communities commonly come together to exercise as a group. Groups have formed that cater to people with diabetes to teach them the best ways for effective and safe exercise. These groups teach the tricks that help eliminate exercise-induced low blood sugar (hypoglycemia). They may encourage weight loss and suggest ways to eat for energy, exercise and diabetes. Joining a group that meets regularly for walking, bike rides or runs will provide motivation to exercise. There may also be understanding, suggestions, support and consolation.

There are many blogs written by and for people with diabetes. They reach out to others who feel ostracized and show the world what a day in the life of someone with diabetes looks like. These can be good resources.

STRESS

Stress can raise blood sugar levels and affect diabetes control (see Figure 1 in Chapter 5). Some major stressors that people with diabetes encounter are:

- discrimination
- uncertainty in whom to tell
- "hiding" diabetes
- handling diabetes at work
- paying for medications

Discrimination

Unfortunately, discrimination against a person with diabetes happens. Fortunately, there are ways to address and deal with a potentially threatening or demeaning person. The Americans with Disabilities Act protects your rights in a work or school environment. Contact a Human Resource (HR) person if coworkers are judgmental or rude, or if the supervisor is limiting job responsibilities without cause or valid justification.

Discrimination sometimes happens when treatment occurs in public, such as when checking a pre-meal blood sugar level or taking pills or insulin while eating out. The best defense against a negative comment from a stranger is a positive attitude. Taking your medicine contributes to a lower HbA1c level. A lower HbA1c level ultimately means fewer or no diabetes-related complications. Remembering this if being discriminated against may be enough to overcome a negative comment.

A different way to address an uncomfortable encounter about diabetes is to have a rehearsed response ready that will address questions while closing the topic. Be firm but not mean. An example might be: "This insulin shot keeps me healthy. I'd rather not talk about it."

Do not avoid public questions or comments by not following a treatment plan. This can lead to high blood sugars, ketones, and, potentially to complications.

Sometimes people are just curious about diabetes and will ask questions if they see a person do a blood sugar check or an insulin shot. This may be an opportunity to educate the person about diabetes. If treatments for diabetes are in an uncomfortable setting, they might need to be administered in a private place. Do not avoid treatments altogether. It is important to keep in mind that informing a co-worker might help in a situation when help is needed (e.g., in the event of low blood sugar levels).

Whom to tell?

Telling people about diabetes can be easy for some and terrifying for others. Acquaintances and co-workers only need to be informed if you choose. Close friends, family and supervisors should at least know what to do in the event of a low blood sugar. If there is a medical emergency related to diabetes, these individuals should know what to do and how to help.

Trusted friends, spouses, significant others and roommates should have more detailed knowledge about the treatment of diabetes. A written emergency plan for those receiving insulin should include the following:

- types of insulin, number of injections, pump usage, etc.

- glucagon instructions for those who use it

- phone numbers of the diabetes providers

- location of supplies

- how to recognize and treat a low or high blood sugar

This information should be easily accessible for them. There are templates or "how to" sheets for low and high blood sugar treatments online. A suggested Emergency Care Plan is included at the end of this chapter. It might be shared with others as seems appropriate.

Financial burdens

Diabetes is a costly disease. Insulin and blood sugar checks may be required daily and even with insurance, co-pays add up. If it looks like the financial responsibilities will be a burden, talk with the diabetes care-provider. Many pharmaceutical companies now have programs that help people without insurance or who have high co-pays to cover the cost of blood sugar strips, insulin or other medical supplies when needed. There may be other options the care team can recommend as well. This might be another topic to discuss with a counselor. Also, certain state and local agencies may have medications available at relatively low cost.

DEPRESSION

Depression is more common in people with type 1 or type 2 diabetes than in the general population. If present, it needs to be addressed and treated or it will interfere with optimal management. Working with a counselor who also has knowledge of diabetes can be very helpful.

EATING DISORDERS

Eating disorders are unfortunately more common in people with diabetes (usually with type 1 diabetes). Anorexia (not eating), bulimia (binging on food followed by self-induced vomiting) and chronic over-eating can occur in people with diabetes. Purposefully missing medications or insulin injections as a weight-loss measure is also a form of an eating disorder. It is found particularly in young women with type 1 diabetes. If these problems are suspected, it is important to seek and receive proper therapy.

SUMMARY

Being diagnosed with diabetes changes a person's life in ways that impact more than just routine lifestyle. Living with diabetes may change the way one perceives oneself and how the person interacts with acquaintances, family, friends and coworkers. Learning how to address the psychological and social impacts of diabetes is an important part of diabetes management.

EMERGENCY CARE PLAN

Health Plan Summary: DIABETES

Name: _____ DOB _____

Home Phone _____

Physician: _____ Phone _____

Fax: _____

Diabetes Educator: _____ Phone _____

Hospital of Choice _____

Emergency Contact Names _____

   and Phone Numbers: _____

Date of Diagnosis _____

Health Concern Diabetes: Type 1 or Type 2: _____

Routine Management Target Blood Sugar Range ___to ___mg/dL (___to ___mmol/L

Required Blood Sugar Checking - Times to Check Blood Sugar:

_____

_____

_____

Diabetes Medications:

❏ Oral diabetes medication(s) Type: _____ Dose: _____

   Time(s) given _____

❏ Oral diabetes medication(s) Type: _____ Dose: _____

   Time(s) given _____

❏ Insulin Type: _____ Dose:_____ Times given: _____

MODERATE LOW BLOOD SUGAR (PERSON IS NOT ALERT):

Symptoms may include combative behavior, being disoriented or incoherent, or having slurred speech.

Treatment of Moderate Low Blood Sugar:

If conscious yet unable to effectively drink the fluids offered:

✔ Administer 3/4 to 1 tube (3 tsp) of glucose gel, or 3/4 tube to 1 tube of cake decorative gel.

✔ Place between cheek and gum then massage into gums, elevate head and encourage swallowing. May be uncooperative.

✔ Retest in 10 minutes. If still below _____ mg/dL (_____mmol/L) re-treat as above.

✔ Give regular snack after retest and when blood sugar rises above _____ mg/dL (_____mmol/L) or when symptoms improve.

Comments: _____

SEVERE LOW BLOOD SUGAR:

Symptoms include: Seizures or loss of consciousness, unable/unwilling to take gel or juice.

Treatment of Severe Low Blood Sugar:

✔ Stay with person ✔ Roll on side ✔ Do not put anything in mouth

✔ Appoint someone to call 911 ✔ Protect from injury ✔ Contact family

✔ Give glucagon: Dose = 1 cc or 100 units (1mg)

Comments: _____

92

PREGNANCY AND DIABETES

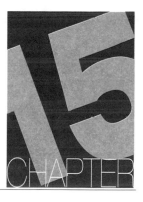

Mary Voelmle, MS, FNP, H. Peter Chase, MD,
Satish K. Garg, MD

PLANNING A PREGNANCY

It is very important to have a visit with your diabetes doctor and your obstetrician at least three months prior to conception. For a woman with diabetes, the best blood sugar control possible without hypoglycemia is most important before and during pregnancy.** Normal or near-normal blood sugar levels reduce the risk of miscarriage and birth defects. Unfortunately, many women with (or without) diabetes do not plan their pregnancies. It is recommended that frequent monitoring of blood sugars and possible use of a continuous glucose monitor (CGM) be started even before pregnancy. Proper planning for pregnancy will result in better HbA1c values prior to pregnancy.

Women with pre-existing diabetes should delay pregnancy until the HbA1c is below 7.0 percent (53 mmol/mol) or until the average blood sugar level is approximately 110 mg/dL (6.1 mmol/L). Folic acid should be taken for three months prior to pregnancy (see "Nutrition and Pregnancy" below). A pre-conception visit with your provider and seeking a high-risk obstetrician are also important.

Many women with type 2 diabetes also have **Polycystic Ovary Syndrome (PCOS)**, another condition associated with insulin resistance and obesity. Women with PCOS may have irregular or infrequent menstrual periods, abnormal reproductive hormones, excess body hair, and infertility. Women with PCOS who are having difficulty becoming pregnant should speak to a reproductive endocrinologist. Weight loss and medications can help improve fertility. Sometimes use of metformin can help with PCOS to help regulate menstrual cycles.

ACHIEVING OPTIMAL GLUCOSE (SUGAR) CONTROL

For people with diabetes, timely intensive management is essential during pregnancy. While some people with type 2 diabetes can manage their blood sugar levels with diet and oral medications, it is often necessary to switch to using insulin to ensure very accurate control for the health of both mother and baby. **Achieving optimal sugar control often involves:**

- frequent blood sugar monitoring (8-10 times daily) or use of a continuous glucose monitor (CGM)

- insulin pump therapy or multiple daily injections (MDI)

- close attention to nutrition

- frequent contact with the healthcare team

Each of these is discussed in more detail below.

BLOOD SUGAR MONITORING/ CONTINUOUS GLUCOSE MONITORING (CGM)

Frequent blood sugar monitoring is essential for optimal glycemic (sugar) control during pregnancy. The suggestions below may be helpful for intensifying blood sugar control.

- Blood sugar and HbA1c goals are given in Table 1.

- It is best to do eight to ten blood sugars per day, before meals and one and two hours after meals as outlined in Table 1 (and/or use a CGM).

- HbA1c levels should be checked monthly until the target level is reached (Table 1), and then every 2-3 months.

- The use of CGM is addressed in Chapter 23.

- Maintaining HbA1c values between 5.0-6.0 percent (31-42 mmol/mol) results in a reduced risk of birth defects in the baby.

- The values one and two hours after meals (Table 1) are important for optimal blood sugar control. Higher blood sugar levels after meals have been associated with big babies and increased complications.

- Take the pre-meal insulin injections 15-20 minutes before meals to prevent post-meal rise in blood sugar levels (discuss with diabetes care-provider).

- Stay in close contact with the healthcare-providers (discussed below). During pregnancy this should be at least weekly.

- Checking blood sugar levels will allow the person to adjust their insulin dosages for different trimesters as sensitivity to insulin changes throughout the pregnancy.

- Nausea is often a problem in early pregnancy. Zofran (8 mg tablets twice daily is often used. However, it is not FDA approved for use in pregnancy.

- Insulin requirements typically increase significantly in the second and third trimesters. Insulin adjustments and frequent blood sugar/CGM monitoring are essential. The insulin dose usually doubles in the third trimester due to the release of steroids from the placenta and an increase in caloric intake.

HIGH BLOOD SUGARS

High blood sugar levels during pregnancy can cause the following:

- an increase in the rate of fetal birth defects (heart, spine, lip, etc), especially during the first trimester

- the birth of larger babies

- an increased risk for injury to both mother and baby during delivery because of the baby's size

- an increase in maternal risk of developing high blood pressure, swelling of feet, and protein leakage in urine (pre-eclampsia), leading to eclampsia or a serious form of pre-eclampsia that may result in liver failure during pregnancy

TABLE 1

Target Values for Blood Sugar and HbA1c Level Before and During Pregnancy*

HbA1c**	<6.0 %***	<42 mmol/mol
	Blood Sugar Levels**	
	mg/dL	mmol/L
Fasting and pre-meal	60-99	3.3-5.4
One hour after meal	<129	<7.3
Two hours after meal	<129	<7.3
2:00 a.m. - 6:00 a.m.	100-130	5.5-7.3

*Per ADA Consensus Statement: *Diabetes Care, 31:1060, 2008*

**If able to be safely achieved.*

***The "<" sign means" less than"*

INSULIN MANAGEMENT

- **Insulin pump therapy** is discussed in detail in Chapter 22. Early use of the pump is often recommended to improve blood sugar control during pregnancy. When possible, it should be initiated before pregnancy.

- **Multiple daily injection (MDI) therapy** involves taking four or more injections of insulin daily. Frequently, NPH (N) insulin is used for the intermediate-acting insulin in MDI. Three or four doses per day (i.e., breakfast, lunch, dinner, snacks) are often used in addition to a rapid-acting insulin such as Humalog, NovoLog, Apidra or Regular (see below). The use of Lantus and Levemir basal insulins is discussed below.

Either method of intensive diabetes management (insulin pump or MDI) is capable of achieving near-normal blood sugar levels. Standard diabetes care (two shots a day) rarely achieves a normal or near-normal HbA1c value and thus should not be a choice during pregnancy. In addition, it may increase the risk of hypoglycemia as insulin dosages may more than double during pregnancy. Basal-bolus insulin therapy is now also frequently used as a form of MDI therapy during pregnancy.

- **Lantus and Levemir** basal insulins have not been properly studied during pregnancy. However, isolated reports of using either insulin during pregnancy with successful outcomes are available. Thus, many physicians now allow patients to continue using their long-acting insulin during pregnancy. Other physicians will change the insulin regimen to use NPH as the basal insulin. As per the FDA label, these insulin analogs are "class 3" for their use during pregnancy. This means their use is considered "off label" during pregnancy.

- **Humalog, NovoLog and Apidra** are rapid (short)-acting insulins that are used for insulin boluses. There are a number of reports on the safety of rapid-acting insulins during pregnancy, and most doctors now recommend their use. Normalizing blood sugar levels after meals is very important. Higher blood sugar levels after meals have been associated with large babies and complications with the pregnancy and delivery. Numerous studies have shown Humalog/NovoLog or Apidra to be more effective for this purpose than Regular insulin. The rapid-acting insulin should ideally be taken 10-20 minutes prior to the time when food is eaten to decrease the post-meal rise in blood sugars. Use of an insulin pen (Chapter 8) is a convenient way to do this for people choosing MDI. Any of these insulins can be used in insulin pumps.

It is important to remember that the post-meal rise in the blood sugar level, especially after one hour, is very important during pregnancy. This occurs because of the increased time to empty the stomach in pregnancy. The rise in blood sugar levels after meals is also in part due to the more rapid absorption of food during pregnancy. Thus, there is a need for an increase in blood sugar monitoring, timing of the rapid-acting insulin injections and appropriate food intake. Most physicians do not use human Regular insulin as a rapid-acting insulin due to its slower onset of action and its inability to effectively reduce post-meal blood sugar levels.

NUTRITION AND PREGNANCY

Nutrition is important during pregnancy and while breastfeeding. Carbohydrate counting and other methods of food management are discussed in Chapter 4. Some specific goals are outlined below.

- It is important to provide adequate calories for maternal and fetal weight gain. This usually involves an additional 300 calories a day during the second and third trimesters and during breastfeeding. One of the frequent questions asked is: "How much weight should I gain?" A 25 to 35 pound (11.4-15.9 kg) weight gain is optimal for a person of normal weight with pregnancy, although this depends greatly on the pre-pregnancy weight. The higher the pre-pregnancy weight, the less that should be gained throughout the pregnancy. Overweight or obese women should not gain more than 25 pounds (11.4 kg) in a singleton pregnancy. Less is acceptable as long as the fetus is growing as it should.

- It is also important to provide adequate vitamins and minerals, including iron and calcium. All women wanting to become pregnant should be certain they are taking 800 µg/day of folic acid, preferably for at least three months prior to pregnancy. This helps to prevent birth defects.

- Alcohol must be avoided to prevent fetal alcohol syndrome and serious congenital defects.

- Not smoking reduces the risk for a premature or low-birth-weight infant.

- Regular meals and snacks are important to prevent hypoglycemia. An evening snack may help to prevent ketones or lows during the night, especially if NPH insulin is being used.

FREQUENT CONTACT WITH THE HEALTHCARE TEAM

Frequent contact with the healthcare-provider is very important in obtaining the best possible sugar control during pregnancy. The suggestions below may be helpful.

- The blood sugar values should be emailed or faxed weekly.

- Clinic visits will vary but are usually monthly or more frequently as needed.

- Medical care from a healthcare-provider with knowledge in the area of diabetes as well as pregnancy is essential.

- Frequent contact with the eye doctor or kidney specialist may also be needed (see below).

PREVENTING ACUTE COMPLICATIONS

High blood sugar was discussed above. Low blood sugars and ketone formation (usually with high blood sugar) are other acute complications.

Low blood sugar (hypoglycemia)

- Frequent blood sugar checking and/or use of a CGM system will help prevent hypoglycemia. However, CGM use has not been approved for use by the FDA during pregnancy, as studies have not yet been done.

- It is well recognized that severe insulin reactions occur more frequently with tight sugar control, especially at night during sleep.

- There has not been evidence that low blood sugars are damaging to the fetus.

- Hypoglycemia is not pleasant for the mom and should be avoided if possible.

Ketones

Ketones usually occur with high blood sugars and are a particular concern during pregnancy.

- Frequent blood sugar checking or CGM use will help to prevent ketone formation and acidosis (Chapter 12).

- Ketones and acidosis may cause miscarriage and are important to avoid. This is particularly important for those using insulin pumps.

When using an insulin pump there is no long-acting insulin and thus, if the infusion catheter is blocked, it may result in high blood sugar levels with ketones and acidosis. Many providers choose to give a small daily dose of a longer-acting insulin like NPH, Levemir or Lantus along with pump usage to avoid or reduce this occurrence. If this is the case, the insulin dose on the pump may need to be adjusted down, especially at night.

- Ketones should be checked anytime the fasting blood sugar is above 240 mg/dL (13.3 mmol/L) or if a random blood sugar level is above 300 mg/dL (16.7 mmol/L).

PREVENTING CHRONIC COMPLICATIONS

Kidney (renal) damage

Kidney damage from diabetes does not usually worsen as a result of pregnancy in women who have normal blood creatinine levels. This is in contrast to the movie "Steel Magnolias." The following list has additional information about pregnancy and the kidneys.

- Women planning a pregnancy should do a urine microalbumin screening and a blood creatinine level prior to pregnancy and after each trimester.

- If the person does have some kidney damage already present, it can worsen with pregnancy.

- If protein is present in the urine, the provider will usually request a 24-hour urine collection for estimation of total protein lost in a day.

- **ACE-inhibitors (see Chapter 16) and cholesterol-lowering agents must be stopped (possible cause of birth defects) in any woman considering pregnancy. Use of other medications should be evaluated after consulting with the care-providers.**

- If blood pressure increases (above 135/85), other medicines such as alpha-methyl dopa (Aldomet®), can be used.

- If kidney concerns are present during pregnancy, clinic visits every two to four weeks may be advised and frequent tests for 24-hour urine collection for protein excretion may be needed.

Eye (retinal) complications

Women who have had diabetes less than five years or who do not have eye (retinal) damage already present, do not usually get eye damage due to pregnancy. They do need their eyes examined prior to the pregnancy and every three months. Additional information related to diabetes pregnancy and the eyes is outlined below.

- If a woman already has moderate eye (retinal) damage from diabetes, this may worsen during pregnancy.

- If control (HbA1c) has not been optimal and improves rapidly, there is an increased risk for eye (retinal) changes. The time interval for visits recommended by a retinal specialist is based on the degree of eye damage.

- Sometimes laser-surgery may be required if eye disease worsens during pregnancy. Very rarely, other surgery may be required for eye damage.

BIRTH

The infant born from a mother with diabetes has an increased risk for low blood sugars as well as for increased size.

- Glucose freely crosses the placenta to the baby resulting in increased insulin output from fetal pancreatic islet cell growth (hyperplasia).

- Due to islet cell hyperplasia (increased size) resulting in increased insulin levels, babies after birth are at a higher risk of developing hypoglycemia (low sugar) and low calcium levels.

- The higher insulin levels in the fetus act as a growth stimulant and result in large babies.

- Over 50 percent of deliveries are vaginal but many times large babies require a cesarean (C-) section. Some obstetricians do not want to take the risk and therefore only do C-sections.

GESTATIONAL DIABETES

Gestational diabetes mellitus (GDM) is diabetes which occurs during pregnancy as a result of insulin resistance due to hormones from the placenta. After diagnosis, the care becomes similar to the care for the person who had diabetes prior to pregnancy. The diagnosis of gestational diabetes has increased significantly in the US, especially in the minorities (Asian, Latino and African-American).

The method for diagnosis of gestational diabetes has been defined by the ADA* and is summarized on the following page.

*ADA, Diabetes Care, 36, Supl 1, S73, 2013

- Perform a 50 or 75 gram oral glucose tolerance test (OGTT), with blood sugar measurements at fasting and at one and two hours, at 24-28 weeks gestation in women not previously diagnosed with diabetes. The OGTT should be performed in the morning after an overnight fast of at least eight hours.

- The diagnosis of GDM is made when any of the blood sugar values are equal or greater than (≥) the following:
  - Fasting ≥92 mg/dL (5.1 mmol/L)**
  - One hr ≥180 mg/dL (10.0 mmol/L)
  - Two hr ≥153 mg/dL (8.5 mmol/L)

Some facts about gestational diabetes are outlined below.

- Regular aerobic exercise and diet may help to lower blood sugar levels before and after meals.

- Gestational diabetes is often associated with weight gain; therefore, losing weight before conception may help to reduce the risk of gestational diabetes.

- Metformin has been used during pregnancy associated with gestational diabetes and appears to be safe.

- Insulin treatment may be necessary; this can be discussed with the diabetes healthcare-provider.

- About 50 percent of women will revert back to normal blood sugar levels after pregnancy, requiring no further treatment. However, these women will have a 50 percent chance of again developing GDM with subsequent pregnancies. In addition, their risk of getting either type 1 or type 2 diabetes is significantly higher than for the general population. This may need to be closely monitored by the healthcare-provider on at least an annual basis.

SUMMARY

When planning a pregnancy, the HbA1c level should be below 7.0 percent (53 mmol/mol) and folic acid supplements should be initiated. High blood sugar levels during pregnancy can lead to birth defects, large babies, and other problems. Frequent communication with the diabetes healthcare-provider is necessary. Proper management of diabetes before and during pregnancy reduces the risk of fetal and maternal complications.

** ≥ sign means greater than or equal to.

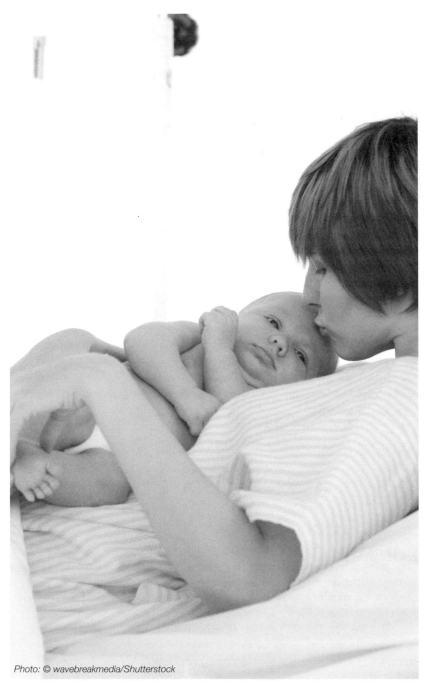

Planning a pregnancy with a visit to your diabetes doctor and obstetrician, and the best sugar control possible before and during the pregnancy, helps result in a healthy, beautiful baby.

MICROVASCULAR COMPLICATIONS (Eye, Kidney and Nerve)

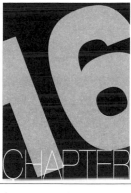

CHAPTER 16

S mall vessels are found all over the body. The small blood vessel (microvascular) complications of diabetes are most commonly found in the eyes (retinopathy), kidneys (nephropathy) and nerves (neuropathy). People with newly diagnosed type 2 diabetes need to be checked for these complications at the time of diagnosis. This is because the diabetes onset is often slow and blood sugar levels may have been elevated for several years prior to diagnosis. People with type 1 diabetes usually have a rapid onset, so checking for complications is usually delayed for several years, depending on glucose control. For people with either type 1 or type 2 diabetes, it is then important to have at least annual screenings for these complications.

RISK FACTORS:

- **Glucose (Sugar) Control:** The risk for diabetes small blood vessel complications are decreased by more than 50 percent with optimal blood glucose (sugar) control. This was shown by the Diabetes Control and Complications Trial (DCCT). The trial also showed that people who had a history of poor sugar control had improvements or slowing of complications when blood sugar levels became better controlled. This means that no matter what the past is for blood sugar levels, better control and more attention to diabetes will always help.

  As discussed in Chapter 2, the HbA1c level is often used as a marker of sugar control. The HbA1c value reflects the attachment of sugar to the red blood cell hemoglobin protein, and is higher when blood sugar levels have been higher. When blood sugar levels are high, the sugar also attaches to other body proteins. These are called AGEs (Advanced Glycation End-products) and are related in part to many of the complications of diabetes.

- **Blood Pressure:** Elevated blood pressure increases the risk for the eye and kidney complications of diabetes. Even mild increases in blood pressure are dangerous.

- **Cholesterol:** Elevated total cholesterol and LDL cholesterol levels are also associated with a higher risk for eye and kidney complications. Increased cholesterol and/or blood pressure may be secondarily associated with kidney disease.

- **Tobacco:** Smoking or chewing tobacco increases the risk for these complications. People with diabetes especially should not smoke or chew tobacco.

EYE COMPLICATIONS

Retinal Changes or Retinopathy

The word retinopathy refers to changes of the retina, which is the layer of tissue at the back of the eye (see picture). This part of the eye has many small blood vessels. Changes in the back of the eye may relate to:

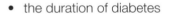

Retina
(back of eye)

Lens

- the duration of diabetes

- the degree of blood sugar control

- increased blood pressure

- tobacco use (makes the changes progress more rapidly)

The DCCT showed that in people without eye changes from diabetes, lower blood sugar levels delayed development of retinopathy by 76 percent. The DCCT also showed that, in people with known early eye changes from diabetes, intensive therapy slowed the progression of retinopathy by 54 percent and reduced the incidence of severe retinopathy by 47 percent.

We do not understand all of the causes of the eye changes of diabetes. There is a small group of people for whom the presence or absence of eye changes seems to not show a relationship to sugar control.

Cataracts

A cataract is a thickening of the lens, which is located at the front of the eye behind the cornea (see picture). Other information about cataracts is summarized below.

- The damage to the lens is believed to be caused by sorbitol, a compound made in the lens from glucose.

- Sorbitol damage occurs when blood sugar levels have been high in the body for a long time.

- Sorbitol in foods is changed by the liver and *does not* cause this damage.

- Damage to the lens can happen at any age.

- Rarely, cataracts can be present at the onset of diabetes if sugar levels have been high for a long time before the diagnosis is made and treatment started.

- Cataracts may show some improvement with optimal sugar control.

- The eye doctor will do a detailed exam for cataracts in the yearly eye exam.

- If cataracts interfere with vision, they can be removed surgically by the eye doctor. Intraocular lens transplants can help to partially restore vision.

KIDNEY DISEASE (DIABETIC NEPHROPATHY)

The kidneys have many important functions in the body.

- They normally filter wastes and water from our blood and make urine.

- When blood sugar levels are high, usually above 180 mg/dL (10 mmol/L), sugar is passed into the urine. When this happens, the pressure is higher in the kidney filtering system (the glomerulus), and changes in the small blood vessels of the kidneys can occur. This increased pressure causes damage to the filtering system so that some proteins start leaking through the filter and appear in the urine.

Kidney disease is one of the most feared of the complications of diabetes and is spoken of as "nephropathy." Nephropathy is more likely to occur in people:

- with type 2 diabetes who have had a delayed diagnosis
- who have had diabetes for a long time
- with high HbA1c values
- with elevated blood pressure
- with high cholesterol levels
- who smoke or chew tobacco

The DCCT showed that improved blood sugar control reduced the occurrence of microalbuminuria (an index of early kidney damage) by 39 percent. Kidney damage (nephropathy, macroalbuminuria) was reduced by 54 percent. It must once again be remembered that inadequate blood sugar control is NOT the only cause of diabetic kidney damage.

Outcomes for kidney disease have improved in people with diabetes in the past few decades. However, serious kidney damage can still occur.

Signs of kidney disease may include:

- increased blood pressure

- ankle swelling, also known as edema (due to fluid collection)

- excessive urine protein spillage

- elevation of the waste materials in the blood (increased blood creatinine and blood urea nitrogen [BUN])

Microalbumin levels

Microalbumin refers to small amounts of albumin, the main protein passing through the kidneys. It is used to detect diabetic kidney damage at an early stage, when it might still be reversible. Microalbumin levels:

- are usually measured on a timed overnight, 24-hour, or "spot" (one-time) urine sample

- should be measured soon after diagnosis for people with type 2 diabetes

- should be measured for people who have had type 1 diabetes for two or more years

- should then be done once yearly so that the interval is not missed when the early damage is still reversible

- are most accurately done by collecting the overnight urine sample (see directions on the next page)

Albumin to creatinine (A/C) ratios:

The albumin to creatinine (A/C) ratio is sometimes used as a convenient screening test, as it can be done on a urine collected in clinic. Unfortunately, they sometimes have false positive results, which then require an overnight or 24 hour urine collection.

MICROALBUMINS

Doctor: _____ Your Name:_____

A. INSTRUCTIONS FOR DOING THE OVERNIGHT URINE COLLECTIONS

COLLECTION #1   DATE: _____

1. Empty your bladder at bedtime and discard this sample.   **TIME:** _____
2. Save **EVERY DROP** of urine during the night.
3. Save **EVERY DROP** of the first morning sample.   **TIME:** _____
   ALL urine from collection #1 should be placed in the same container.
4. Measure the volume of the urine sample.   **TOTAL VOLUME:** _____

COLLECTION #2   DATE: _____

1. Empty your bladder at bedtime and discard this sample.   **TIME:** _____
2. Save **EVERY DROP** of urine during the night.
3. Save **EVERY DROP** of the first morning sample.   **TIME:** _____
   ALL urine from collection #2 should be placed in the same container.
4. Measure the volume of the urine sample.   **TOTAL VOLUME:** _____

B. DIRECTIONS FOR MEASURING THE VOLUME

1. Have a measuring cup or (better) a cylinder - preferably marked in cc (ml). One cup is 240cc. Urine is sterile and it is ok to use cooking measuring cups (just wash prior to next use for cooking).

2. Measure the total cc of each overnight sample and put the amounts in the blanks for step 4 for collections #1 and #2.

3. Put a sample of each urine collection in a clean tube. The rest may be discarded. Any clean red top tube from a doctor's office, clinic or hospital lab will work. Label which sample (#1 or #2) it is, put your name on the tube, and put the tube in a cup in the refrigerator until you get to your clinic. Remember to bring this sheet with the times and total volumes with you.

C. IMPORTANT INFORMATION ABOUT YOUR COLLECTIONS

1. Label each tube with your name and #1 or #2.

2. You may use any CLEAN container you have at home that will not leak to collect the sample. Containers may not be provided.

3. Store the tubes of urine in the refrigerator until your visit (samples are good for one week if kept cold).

4. DO NOT mix collections #1 and #2 together in the same container.

5. DO NOT drink caffeinated or alcoholic beverages or use tobacco after 10 p.m. the evening of the collections.

6. DO NOT exercise strenuously for the four hours prior to bedtime.

7. DO NOT collect specimens during a menstrual period.

8. Failure to follow directions exactly may cause incorrect results.

9. If you have any questions, please call your healthcare-provider.

Some facts about elevated microalbumin levels are outlined below.

- A "borderline microalbumin level" for timed overnight urine collections is a value between 7.6 µg/minute and 20 µg/minute. This "borderline" range represents a time period when optimal sugar and/or blood pressure control may help to lower the value or keep it from going higher.

- Medications are not usually given for a "borderline" level, as it may still be possible to return the value to normal by lowering the HbA1c.

- If the urine microalbumin value is between 20 and 300 µg/minute, it is called "**micro**albuminuria" and may still be reversible with lowering of blood sugar values, blood pressure control and medications (ACE-inhibitor, see below). Generally, two of three samples above 20 µg/min are required prior to diagnosis.

- Some providers initiate the treatment with ACE-inhibitors once multiple microalbumin levels are significantly higher (above 10 µg/min), or as a preventative measure even without any evidence of protein spillage in the urine. However, there is little data to suggest that using these medications before the onset of kidney disease actually prevents nephropathy. There may be other benefits for using ACE-inhibitors such as reducing blood pressure, heart disease, and/or decreasing the chance of neuropathy.

- Protein intake may need to be reduced based on the level of kidney or eye disease. This is true for anyone who has microalbumin levels above 20 micrograms/minute, but particularly for those who have levels above 300 micrograms/minute (nephropathy or **macro**albuminuria).

Collection of the proper samples for microalbumin determinations is an important part of diabetes management.

- It is up to the person and the physician to make sure that the urine collections to detect kidney changes are done at the recommended times.

- If the person is unable to collect an overnight urine as described in this chapter, bringing in a portion of the first morning urine is second best. This provides a urine sample from when the person slept. It avoids the 10-14 percent false positives that occur with collecting a random sample in the clinic.

- For a random, non-timed urine, a concentration of greater than 30 micrograms of albumin per mg of creatinine is considered to be "microalbuminuria." This indicates the need for the overnight or the 24-hour urine collection to be done.

The past three decades have brought significant advances in the prevention, detection and treatment of diabetic kidney damage.

- If the microalbumin level on the overnight or the 24-hour urine sample is high, medicines may be effective in reversing or slowing the kidney damage.

- The usual medicine that is tried first is an **ACE-inhibitor (ACE = A**ngiotensin-**C**onverting **E**nzyme). These medications prevent formation of angiotensin II, which is a very potent constrictor of blood vessels. The result is less pressure buildup in the kidneys. There are several ACE-inhibitors, all of which are probably effective if given in adequate dosage. Another similar class of medications are called **ARBs** (or **A**ngiotensin **R**eceptor **B**lockers). These are particularly helpful when a cough or other side effects occur from the use of an ACE-inhibitor. Your healthcare-provider will choose the appropriate medication. Occassionally, both ACE and ARBs are needed to control kidney damage and blood pressure.

- Early kidney damage is detectable and methods to reverse or slow down kidney damage are available. This has now resulted in a decline in the incidence of kidney failure from diabetes.

NEUROPATHY (NERVE DAMAGE)

Diabetic neuropathy, or "damage to the nerves," is a condition usually seen in people who have had very high sugar levels for a long time. It is also sometimes present at diagnosis in people with type 2 diabetes who have had high sugar levels for a prolonged period before diagnosis.

Neuropathy is a complex condition that we still do not completely understand. The DCCT found that the incidence of neuropathy was 60 percent less in the group with lower blood sugar levels. As with cataracts, neuropathy is believed to be related, at least in part, to increased sorbitol levels deposited in the nerves. The sorbitol is made from sugar. There is also a decrease in another compound (myoinositol) which is important for the nerves. Symptoms can include numbness, tingling, sharp pains in the lower legs or feet (sometimes referred to as "stocking" or "glove" paresthesia or anesthesia). In men, erectile dysfunction (ED) is at least partly due to nerve damage. It may respond to medications (Cialis®, Viagra®, etc.), erection aids (e.g., vacuum devices) and/or other therapy. Much research is being done to find new and better medications for the treatment of neuropathy.

"Sympathetic" or "Autonomic" Neuropathy

This type of neuropathy can affect any of the organs inside the body. The most frequent involves the gastrointestinal tract ("gastroparesis"). The stomach cannot empty normally, and may pass the food from the stomach rapidly. It may result in bloating and/or vomiting. The help of a knowledgeable gastroenterologist should be sought. Small, frequent meals and medications are sometimes helpful.

SUMMARY

Better sugar, blood pressure, and cholesterol management, as well as stopping or avoiding smoking, have resulted in a lower incidence of the eye, kidney and nerve complications of diabetes. Regular screening for complications can allow early treatment to reverse or slow damage. Timely clinic visits are an important part of prevention.

MACROVASCULAR COMPLICATIONS

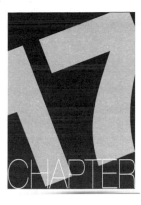

Erin C. Cobry, MD, H. Peter Chase, MD, Satish K. Garg, MD

Macrovascular is a term used to refer to the medium to large blood vessels in the body. With diabetes, there is a risk of developing complications related to these blood vessels. The cardiovascular (heart/blood vessel) system and the extremities, especially the feet, take precedence in people with diabetes. The risk factors for macrovascular complications are similar to those discussed previously in Chapter 16 for the microvascular complications. They are summarized in the box below.

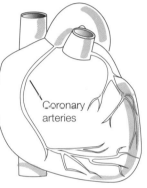

Coronary arteries

Risk Factors	Aim for Cardiovascular Complications Prevention
glucose (sugar) control	HbA1c below 7.0% (53 mmol/mol)
blood pressure	below 130/80
tobacco use	don't use
elevated total cholesterol,	below 200 mg/dL (5.2 mmol/L)
elevated LDL-cholesterol	below 100 mg/dL (2.6 mmol/L)
elevated (fasting) triglyceride	below 150 mg/dl (1.7 mmol/L)

If any of the levels are elevated, it is important to discuss with your physician. In addition, the presence of kidney disease worsens the above risk factors for cardiovascular disease. These are all discussed below and relate to both type 1 and type 2 diabetes.

PREVENTION

Glycemic (Sugar) Control

The best way to decrease the macrovascular complications is to prevent or reverse type 2 diabetes. This is discussed in Chapters 2 (Pre-Type 2 Diabetes), 4, 5, 6 and 18. Many studies have shown that blood sugar control is very closely related to vascular disease. The measures discussed throughout this book can result in better sugar control and a lower risk for most diabetes complications, including macrovascular problems. This is true for people who have type 2 or type 1 diabetes.

Blood Pressure

While blood sugar control is very important for decreasing the risk of complications, there are other factors that play a role, including high blood pressure. Elevated blood pressure over a period of time causes damage to all of the body's blood vessels. Close follow up with your physician and adherence to treatment is essential. If necessary, there are many different types of medications that can be used to help lower blood pressure. The first one usually added for a person with diabetes (type 2 or type 1) is an ACE-Inhibitor (discussed previously in Chapter 16). This is because of the beneficial effects on the kidneys as well as the ability to lower blood pressure.

Tobacco Use

Many studies have shown a strong link between smoking and cardiovascular disease. Smoking is not recommended for anyone, especially for people with type 1 or type 2 diabetes. This is due to both the microvascular and macrovascular complications that are associated with tobacco use.

Elevated Blood Lipids

Elevated total cholesterol, triglycerides, and LDL (low density lipoprotein) cholesterol all add to blood vessel atherosclerosis (hardening of the arteries). There are some genetic (familial) factors that contribute to elevations in cholesterol. Improving blood sugar control will often improve the lipid profile. The blood lipid levels are also affected by eating high fat meals (Chapter 3). People with type 1 or type 2 diabetes should have their blood lipid levels checked annually. If elevations are present, behavioral and/or medical treatment should be initiated. Management usually starts with dietary changes, as described in Chapter 3, with the later addition of medications as needed. The main class of medications used for treatment is the

HMG-CoA reductase inhibitors, commonly known as "statins." They block the body's ability to make cholesterol. Generic forms of this medicine are now available at greatly reduced costs.

CARDIOVASCULAR DISEASE

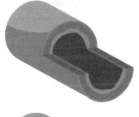

Normal cross section of artery

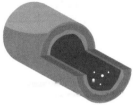

Cholesterol particles

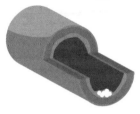

A plaque forms in the artery (partial block)

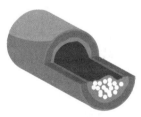

Artery becomes narrowed and may become completely blocked, usually due to a hemorrhage within the plaque.

The term "cardiovascular" refers to the system involving the heart and medium- and large-sized blood vessels. More adults with diabetes die of cardiovascular complications than of any other cause. Lipid (fat) is deposited along the walls of the blood vessels and becomes calcified (hardened) over time. This then results in a blockage of the blood flow through the blood vessels. The thickening of the blood vessel wall is called 'atherosclerosis.' Atherosclerosis can occur in any of the arteries supplying blood to the heart or to the rest of the body. However, the blood vessels that supply blood to the heart, brain and extremities are of most concern in people with diabetes.

Illustration: © GRei/Shutterstock

Heart (Angina, Heart Attack)

If the blood flow through the coronary arteries is blocked, the following may occur:

- no symptoms ("silent" or "asymptomatic"), especially if neuropathy and an inability to feel pain is also present
- chest pain – particularly pain that spreads to the left shoulder, arm or jaw (the latter especially in women). Women often have less specific symptoms and are sometimes harder to diagnose.
- tightness of the chest or the feeling of 'pressure' on the chest wall
- shortness of breath or breathing difficulty with minimal exercise, such as walking short distances

When these symptoms occur, it is important to call 911 or to head to an emergency room immediately. If the blockage is partial ("angina"), resting or medications (such as aspirin or nitroglycerin) may help with the pain. Depending on the extent of the block, surgery may also be necessary to open up the blockage. If there is no blood flow through the arteries providing blood to an area in the heart (a "heart attack"), surgery is commonly needed if the person's condition is stable enough.

Brain (Stroke, Transient Ischemic Attack [TIA])

A stroke is caused by rapid changes in the supply of the blood to the brain. Blockage of the blood vessel and blood flow (ischemia) to a portion of the brain is one cause of stroke.

The other major cause is from a hemorrhage or bleed. Partial and temporary blockage is called a **transient ischemic attack (TIA)** in which the symptoms typically resolve quickly without long-term complications.

Symptoms of a stroke can vary based on the artery blocked, but may include some transient or permanent neurological deficit like:

- facial drooping
- slurred speech or inability to talk
- weakness on one side of the body
- loss of balance or falling
- changes in vision

A stroke or TIA is a medical emergency and must be treated immediately to prevent permanent damage to the brain. There are treatments available that can be used to reverse the symptoms if it is diagnosed quickly enough. If the source of the stroke is a clot of blood from the arteries in the neck, surgery may be needed to remove the blockage and prevent a future stroke.

Lower Extremities

The lower extremities arc particularly affected in people with type 2 diabetes. They are the farthest from the heart and often have poor circulation. The term "peripheral artery disease" (PAD) is often used. Any atherosclerosis (thickening of the arteries and decrease in blood supply) will worsen the circulation. If neuropathy (Chapter 16) is also present, the person may not feel pain with injuries, leading to wounds that are not recognized and not treated.

Symptoms of blockage of lower-extremity blood vessels might include the following:

- cramping with walking ("intermittent claudication")
- sores on the legs or feet that do not heal so that seeking medical attention is necessary
- numbness or weakness in the leg
- coldness in the leg or foot, especially when compared to the other leg
- changes in the color of the leg or foot
- hair loss on the leg

Common treatments beyond improving sugar control may include:

- treatment with statins to lower blood lipids (cholesterol, LDL)
- medicines to lower blood pressure
- stopping smoking/tobacco use
- aspirin or other blood thinners (e.g., Plavix®)

If the blockage of the blood vessels is severe, surgery or medications may be helpful and necessary. Unfortunately, if the blockage becomes complete and there is very little to no blood flow, the tissue may not survive and amputation of a toe, foot or leg may be required.

Diabetes is the leading cause of amputations in the U.S. due to the combination of decreased blood flow to the limb as well as the inability to feel when an injury occurs. As a result, proper treatment is often not initiated.

SUMMARY

The medium and large vessel complications of diabetes can be devastating. This is true for both type 1 and type 2 diabetes. The macrovascular effects are not usually seen for years following the onset of the diabetes and as a result are often forgotten or not taken seriously. It is very important that optimal blood sugar control be maintained from the beginning to prevent complications in later years. It is also important to be closely followed by a healthcare-provider to have routine evaluations done, including cholesterol levels, blood pressure checks and HbA1c measurements.

RESEARCH AND TYPE 2 DIABETES

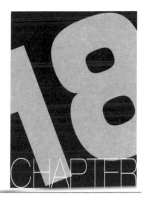

PATHOPHYSIOLOGY OF TYPE 2 DIABETES

Type 2 diabetes is progressive in nature and has multiple factors contributing to its cause. An important risk factor is being **overweight or obese**. This results in the body needing to increase insulin output from the beta cells in the pancreas. The pancreas cannot continue to produce more insulin, and thus the blood sugar levels rise.

Another important factor in type 2 diabetes is the **decrease in insulin sensitivity (insulin resistance)**. Lack of exercise contributes to insulin resistance. This further contributes to the need for elevated levels of insulin production from the pancreas and later results in high blood sugar levels. In most instances, elevations in blood sugar levels are initially detected after meals (also resulting in slight elevations in HbA1c levels). Early type 2 diabetes can be detected by doing an oral glucose tolerance test (OGTT), which has been discussed in Chapter 2. In the later stages of the disease, fasting blood sugar levels also rise, resulting in significant elevations of HbA1c values.

In the majority of patients with type 2 diabetes, the **classical symptoms** of polyuria (frequent urination), polydipsia (frequent drinking) and polyphagia (frequent eating) are absent due to the gradual onset. It is important that the disease is detected early so that complications can be minimized. At the time of diagnosis, early complications may already be present (e.g., cataracts, change in vision, or loss of sensation in hands and feet [diabetic neuropathy]). **On average, a patient may have higher blood sugar levels for five to ten years before they are diagnosed. It should be clear that the best approach to type 2 diabetes is to prevent or delay the onset of the disease.**

PREVENTION RESEARCH

A large study called The Diabetes Prevention Program (DPP) studied over 3,000 people with pre-type 2 diabetes*. Data from three groups (lifestyle intervention, metformin treatment, and controls) was analyzed. People in the lifestyle intervention arm of the study used a low-fat, reduced-calorie food program and exercised a minimum of 150 minutes per week. The initial aim was to reduce body weight by at least seven percent. Progression to diabetes was initially reduced by more than half compared to randomized controls (people not receiving treatment). Even after ten years, the likelihood of getting diabetes was reduced by 34 percent. Another group of people in the study received the medicine, metformin. They had an initial reduction of getting diabetes by 31 percent, which was still reduced by 18 percent after ten years. People in the study, regardless of their treatment group, who converted their sugar metabolism to normal either one, two or three times during the study had respectively, a 41, 61 and 67 percent lower likelihood of progressing to diabetes. There are now so many people in the world who have *pre-type 2 diabetes, more than a half-billion, that halting its progression **must** be an essential focus* of research in the next decade. Risk factors for type 2 diabetes are discussed below.

The incidence of type 2 diabetes is also increasing in teenagers. Beginning screening and interventions in childhood and adolescence will help to prevent childhood obesity and early onset type 2 diabetes. Interventions in childhood and adolescence to lose weight and maintain healthy diets and exercise programs may be beneficial in preventing, or at least delaying, the onset of type 2 diabetes later in life.

RISK FACTORS RESEARCH

Risk factors for developing type 2 diabetes have been studied extensively in recent years, and will continue to receive emphasis. Factors identified to date include the following:

- a close relative with type 2 diabetes

- lack of life-style changes, including less than 90 minutes per week of exercise and eating a high calorie, high fat diet

- excessive intake of sugar-sweetened drinks

- over 45 years old

- BMI over 25 kg/m^2 (overweight) or especially over 35 kg/m^2 (obesity)

- for Asians, lower BMI levels might indicate overweight and obesity

- metabolic syndrome (see Chapter 2)

Diabetes Prevention Program Research Group, NEngl J Med, 346-393, 2002

- high abdominal fat (waist measurement at navel [belly button] above 40 inches [100cm])**

- non-Caucasian, especially African-American, Latino, American Indian and Asian-American

- HDL level below 35 mg/dL (0.9 mmol/L)

- triglyceride level above 250 mg/dL (2.82 mmol/L)

- women who delivered a baby weighing over nine pounds or who had gestational diabetes

- women with polycystic ovary syndrome (see Chapter 15)

- borderline elevated HbA1c level (e.g., 6.0-6.4 percent [42-46 mmol/mol])

It is currently recommended that all adults who are overweight (BMI above 25 kg/m²), and who have one or more of the other risk factors, be screened for type 2 diabetes (see Diagnosis and Laboratory Tests, Chapter 2).

Genes are being identified that put people at an increased risk for developing type 2 diabetes, high blood cholesterol or heart disease. Currently there are 16 genes that have been found to be associated with type 2 diabetes. At this time, routine genetic screening is not recommended. However, at some point in the future it might be possible to determine people who are at an unusually high risk for developing type 2 diabetes based on their genetics. Given the ability to adjust lifestyle issues before the disease is diagnosed, it might be possible to prevent the disease in people with high genetic risk.

There are also significant dietary risk factors that increase the chance of developing type 2 diabetes. Studies have shown that regular consumption of sugar-sweetened drinks (including fruit juices, sweetened teas, sodas, and sports or energy drinks) in both adults and children leads not only to obesity but also to type 2 diabetes. In one study, done by Dr. Frank Hu at Harvard, people drinking between one to two 12 ounce servings per day increased their risk of developing type 2 diabetes by 26 percent when compared to people who drank less than one sugar drink per month. Recommendations are to decrease the number of sugar beverages and replace them with healthier choices, such as water.

*_*Others recommend taking a measurement (parallel to the floor) at the top of the hip bone. Men should be below 40 inches (102 cm) and women below 35 inches (88 cm). It is the fat inside the abdomen (fisceral fat) that is most important. Waist measurement is a rough measurement of visceral fat._

The more risk factors a person has, the greater the likelihood of developing type 2 diabetes. Identification of risk factors can help in preventing type 2 diabetes. If the diabetes can be prevented, secondary complications such as cardiovascular disease (Chapter 17) will also be reduced.

Risk factors will continue to be studied in future years. Different genetic alterations are currently receiving much emphasis. Environmental pollutants are also being evaluated.

MEDICATION RESEARCH

Because type 2 diabetes is so prevalent and is increasing greatly, every major pharmaceutical company would like to have the newest, latest, and best medicine.

Weight Loss Medications:

Recent studies are showing help in weight-loss from medications when food plans and exercise are unsuccessful. Two medicines for weight loss have been approved by the FDA:

1) Phentermine/topiramate ER (extended release) (Qsymia®)

2) Lorcaserin (Belviq®)

These medications have side effects and should be administered by a physician knowledgeable in their use and contraindications. Qsymia must not be taken if there is any chance of pregnancy (high risk for birth defects). Long term safety data is not yet available. In addition, they are only effective if the person is also motivated to make lifestyle corrections.

Recent New Diabetes Medications:

Over the past decade, many new classes of diabetes medications have been developed. These include new insulins, GLP analogs, and DPP4 inhibitors (all discussed in Chapter 6). Other recent medications include alpha glucosidase inhibitors (Acarbose), amylin analogs (Symlin®), meglitinides, and thiozolodinediones.

Canagliflozin (Invokana®), a sodium glucose co-transporter-2 (SGLT2) inhibitor, has recently been approved by the FDA to reduce high blood sugar levels. It works by increasing urinary sugar excretion. There has also been some effect in reducing sugar absorption in the intestine. It also decreases blood pressure and weight. The major side effect to date has been genital and urinary tract infections (15 percent rate in women and nine percent in men). Continued research for possible cardiovascular complications is required.

Metformin helps in losing weight. It is important to keep side effects in mind while taking these medications (see Chapter 6).

Novel Approaches in Development

Research is also being done on the following novel approaches to treat diabetes:

- Researching alternative ways to deliver insulin may eliminate the need for injections. These may include inhaled insulin, oral insulin, or insulin that is absorbed through the skin.

- "Smart" insulins are being developed which automatically adjust doses when blood sugar levels are high or low.

- The use of dopamine stimulators helps to roduce the amount of sugar released from the livor after meals. Bromocriptine (Cycloset®) is currently an approved medication in this category, and research will likely discover others.

- The use of bile acid sequesterants (e.g., Colesevelam) helps to control both blood sugar and lipid levels.

Overall, the important message is that new medicines continue to be developed for the treatment of type 2 diabetes.

RESEARCH ON THE TREATMENT OF COMPLICATIONS

Delayed wound healing is a common complication in people with diabetes. New research is being done to determine a way to speed the wound healing process and therefore prevent the risk of infection, amputation and even death. Molecules that lead to the growth of cells in the skin and blood vessels are being studied. By increasing the flow of blood to the wound, the skin and tissue will be able to receive the nutrients needed to heal properly and quickly.

TYPES OF STOMACH SURGERY USED TO PREVENT OR REVERSE TYPE 2 DIABETES

Much research is being reported relating to the two main types of stomach surgery used to prevent or reverse type 2 diabetes. The two main types of surgery are stomach banding and the Roux-en-Y (bypass) procedure. Both have been used primarily in obese people who are physically, emotionally or medically unable to perform exercise and diet modifications to result in significant weight loss.

Stomach (Gastric) Banding:

In this surgical procedure (Figure 1), a band is placed around the upper stomach to reduce the amount of food the stomach can hold. It can be done with a small abdominal incision, a laparoscopic procedure, which generally takes about an hour. The band can later be tightened or loosened depending on the person's needs. It generally results in the person eating less food. The procedure is more apt to be used for patients who are motivated, have a BMI of 40 or less and are high-risk patients, or those who fear more invasive (e.g., gastric bypass) surgery. Weight loss is often modest (20-30 pounds or 9-14 kg) and it requires changing eating habits at the same time or the weight will be gained back. Results are now being reported in relation to prevention of diabetes, as well as for the reversal of diabetes in those who already have it (see below).

FIGURE 1

Stomach (Gastric) Banding

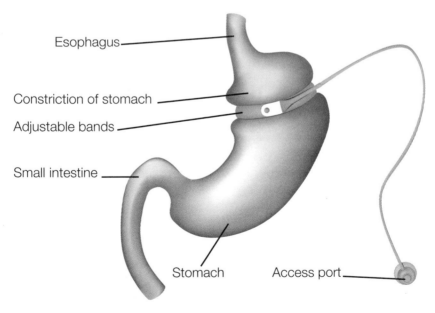

Illustration: © Alila Medical Images/Shutterstock

Gastric (Stomach) Bypass (Roux-en-Y or Sleeve) Surgery:

This procedure involves removing the stomach from active use. Essentially, the swallowing tube (esophagus) is attached directly to the small intestine (Figure 2). It is usually done during open surgery or through a small incision using a laparoscope. It is a more extensive procedure than gastric banding, and the length of surgery is usually three to four hours. Results using this surgical procedure for the prevention or reversal of diabetes are described below.

FIGURE 2
Stomach Bypass Surgery

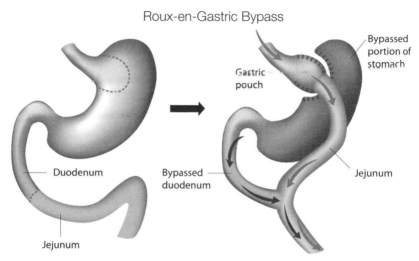

Illustration: © Alila Medical Images/Shutterstock

SURGERY AND THE PREVENTION OF DIABETES

There are now several reports of gastric (stomach) surgery in obese adults resulting in the prevention of type 2 diabetes. A large study was described from Sweden* in which 1,658 non-diabetic obese adults received either banding or bypass surgery (no differences in results) versus 1,771 controls who received the usual weight loss management. During follow-up, type 2 diabetes developed in 392 of the control subjects (28 percent), compared to only 110 (7 percent) of the surgery subjects. In addition, for those who had borderline abnormal blood sugar levels, there was an even greater

*Carlsson, LMS et al., N Engl J. Med. 367, 695-704, 2012;
Sjoholm et. al., Diabetes Care 36, 1335, 2013

(87 percent) risk reduction for developing diabetes. The stomach surgery group had lost about 20 kg (44 pounds) after both 10 and 15 years, whereas the control group had no change in body weight. Three patients (0.2 percent) died within 90 days of the surgery and 46 (2.6 percent) had complications requiring repeat surgery. Thus, although the risk is now less after years of experience, the surgery does have potential complications. It is obviously impractical to consider gastric surgery for the millions of obese adults. However, it may be the treatment of choice for some individuals.

SURGERY AND THE REVERSAL OF DIABETES

A research report by Dr. Sarah Steven from Newcastle, England in 2012 described 73 patients with type 2 diabetes who had the Roux-en-Y gastric bypass surgery. Her patients were obese (mean BMI of 50 kg/M^2) and had diabetes for a mean of five years. They were receiving metformin and sometimes other oral medications and 12 received insulin. She reported that diabetes was reversed with no medications required in 73 percent of patients who had diabetes less than four years. For those who had diabetes for over eight years, 21 percent no longer needed any diabetes medications. The most important factor in reversal of diabetes was clearly the amount of weight lost.

SUMMARY

The prevalence of type 2 diabetes continues to rise. Prevention of type 2 diabetes is one of the most important issues in medicine at this time and is a very active field for studies. It may be accomplished with early diagnosis, lifestyle intervention, medications, or surgery. The continued development of new medications to prevent and/or treat type 2 diabetes and its complications is also an important area for research.

INTRODUCTION: TYPE 1 DIABETES

Much of the education for type 1 diabetes is similar to that for type 2 diabetes. It is not necessary to repeat previous chapters. The suggested reading order for learning about type 1 diabetes, based on the necessities of management, is outlined below.

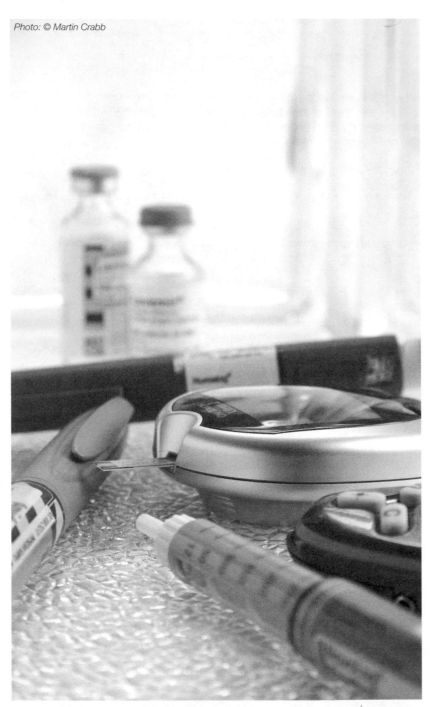

Blood sugar checking is important for people with diabetes who take insulin.

WHAT IS TYPE 1 DIABETES? Causes, Symptoms and Diagnosis

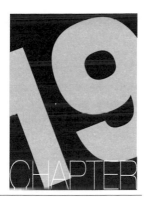

CHAPTER 19

CAUSES

Type 1 diabetes is caused by a combination of an inherited **genetic** risk, an **environmental** factor and an **autoimmune reaction** ("self-allergy"). The environmental cause is unknown, although some doctors think this agent may be a virus infection and/or something in the diet. With an autoimmune disease, the body's immune system mistakenly attacks its own healthy cells. When this happens, antibodies are made against specific cells in the body. In this case it is against the islet cells in the pancreas where insulin is made, and **islet cell antibodies** result. There are neither autoimmune reactions nor islet cell antibodies in people who have type 2 diabetes.

Insulin is a hormone which allows sugar to pass from the blood into body cells to be used for energy. As the autoimmune reaction progresses against the islet cells in the pancreas, less and less insulin is made (Figure 1). As insulin production decreases, less sugar passes into the body's cells for energy and the blood sugar levels rise. For the purposes of this book, the words "sugar" and "glucose" are used interchangeably. In the scientific world, the term "sugar" includes many different types, not just glucose.

SYMPTOMS

The symptoms of type 1 diabetes are due to elevated blood sugar levels, and may thus be the same for both type 1 and type 2 diabetes. They are usually more prominent in people presenting with type 1 diabetes. The symptoms may include any of the following:

- frequent urination (polyuria), often most noticeable at night
- increased thirst (polydipsia)
- eating more and still feeling hungry (polyphagia)
- weight loss
- less energy

- headaches
- blurred vision

Some people don't have any symptoms when diagnosed. This is especially true early in the type 1 diabetes autoimmune process. These people are sometimes diagnosed by a high blood sugar level that is measured on a routine physical exam. Others are diagnosed when they have a high blood sugar level on a test called an Oral Glucose Tolerance Test (OGTT) as discussed Chapter 2.

The cause of frequent urination is because the high blood sugar causes sugar to pass from the blood through the kidneys into the urine. Water goes out with the sugar, so urination is increased. Frequent drinking of fluids then occurs to replace the water lost as a result of the frequent urination. Weight loss is because the body cannot use sugar for energy due to a lack of insulin activity. Body fat and protein are then broken down for energy.

More people who develop type 1 diabetes are now being found to be overweight at the time of diagnosis. Others gain excessive weight after treatment is begun. As a result, insulin resistance as in type 2 diabetes may be present.

DIAGNOSIS

Pre-diabetes

For people with pre-type 1 diabetes, the diagnosis is based on 'borderline' blood sugar levels (Table 1, Chapter 2) and any positive islet cell antibodies (see below). The sugar levels are above normal, but are not yet in the range to diagnose diabetes. The presence of the antibodies shows that the islet cells in the pancreas (where insulin is made) have been injured. An autoimmune process ("self-allergy") is underway and type 1 diabetes is the culprit. Antibodies do not occur with type 2 diabetes.

Relatives of people with type 1 diabetes are often screened for the islet cell antibodies (see Chapter 24). One or more pancreas islet auto-antibodies (GAD, ICA512, insulin and/or ZnT8) may be present in the blood of people with type 1 diabetes or pre-type 1 diabetes. The most common positive autoantibody for adults diagnosed with type 1 diabetes, or with Latent-Autoimmune Diabetes in Adults (LADA), is the GAD autoantibody.

Diabetes

In order to be diagnosed with diabetes, one of the following conditions must be met:

- fasting blood sugar level above 126 mg/dL (7.0 mmol/L)
- blood sugar level above 200 mg/dL (11.1 mmol/L) at two hours in an OGTT (see below)
- random blood sugar(s) above 200 mg/dL (11.1 mmol/L) and symptoms of diabetes
- HbA1c above 6.5 percent (48 mmol/mol)

Table 1 in Chapter 2 compares the normal, pre-diabetic, and diabetic ranges of both blood sugar levels and HbA1c values. The two-hour **oral glucose tolerance test (OGTT)** is a tool often used to help diagnose diabetes. The first blood sugar level is done after fasting (no food for eight hours). After the fasting blood sugar is drawn, the person drinks a high sugar drink (e.g., Glucola™) within five minutes. A second blood sample is drawn after two hours. Sometimes the diagnosis is made on the basis of symptoms and elevated blood sugar levels (above 200 mg/dL or 11.1 mmol/L). If this is the case, the OGTT is not needed.

The other diagnostic test is the **hemoglobin A1c level** (**HbA1c,** often called the "**A1c**"). Sugar in the blood attaches to the hemoglobin protein in red blood cells to form HbA1c (see Figure 2 in Chapter 2).

The HbA1c level reflects how often the blood sugars have been high in the past two to three months. The HbA1c level is higher when the blood sugars have been higher. The non-diabetic HbA1c level is usually below 6.0 percent (42 mmol/mol). Six to 6.5 percent (42 to 48 mmol/mol) may indicate pre-diabetes. The American Diabetes Association (ADA) considers a value above 6.5 percent (48 mmol/mol) to be diagnostic of diabetes. Table 1 may help people relate their HbA1c level to an average blood sugar level over the past three months.

Blood sugar and HbA1c values are used to diagnose both pre-diabetes and diabetes. They are also used for the diagnosis of both type 1 and type 2 diabetes. The major difference is the usual presence of islet cell antibodies in the blood of people who have type 1 diabetes. Islet cell antibodies are not present in the blood of people who have type 2 diabetes.

SUMMARY

Type 1 and type 2 diabetes have different causes. Although both have a genetic (inherited) part, type 1 is partly autoimmune and type 2 is usually associated with being overweight. The same tests are used in diagnosing both types of diabetes. The symptoms may also be the same in both conditions. However, type 2 diabetes usually progresses slowly over a longer period of time prior to the diagnosis and has fewer symptoms. In contrast, the onset of type 1 diabetes usually happens over a shorter time period and often has more symptoms just prior to diagnosis.

FIGURE 1

The Gradual Onset of Type 1 Diabetes

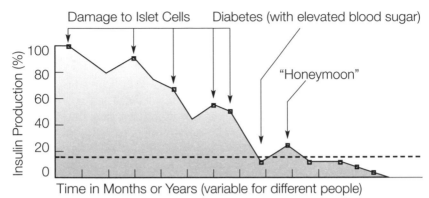

It is now believed that diabetes develops gradually, over many months or many years. It does not just come on suddenly in the week or two before the elevated blood sugars. Many insults (represented by the arrows in this Figure) likely result in further damage until the diagnosis of diabetes is made. The insults may include viral infections, stress, parts of the diet, or other agents. These agents may work by "activating" white blood cells in the islets to make toxic chemicals that cause injury to the insulin-producing cells (beta cells). However, a "genetic-predisposition" (inherited factors) must be present for the process to start.

TABLE 1

Correlation of HbA1c with Estimated Average Blood Sugar Levels

HbA1c			Mean blood sugar	
%	mmol/mol		mg/dL	mmol/L
6	42	→	126	7.0
7	53	→	154	8.6
8	64	→	192	10.2
9	75	→	212	11.8
10	86	→	240	13.4
11	97	→	269	14.9
12	108	→	298	16.5

Taken in part from: American Diabetes Association, Diabetes Care 2011; 36 (suppl 1): S18
In the U.S., HbA1c is usually reported as a percent and blood sugar in mg/dL. Many other countries use mmol/mol and mmol/L, respectively, for the two measurements.

TREATMENT OF TYPE 1 DIABETES

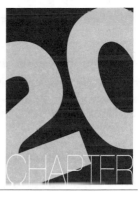

Most of the therapies for type 1 diabetes are similar to those already described for type 2 diabetes, particularly for the later stages when insulin injections are needed. A suggested reading order for learning about type 1 diabetes is outlined on page 125. Many of the subjects reviewed here are discussed in more detail in earlier chapters, and the chapter numbers are listed. A synopsis *First Book for Understanding Diabetes* and a larger book, *Understanding Diabetes*, focus on type 1 diabetes and are available for those who would like more information (see back for ordering information).

INSULIN THERAPY

Insulin therapy is different for people with type 1 diabetes in that insulin treatment begins on the day of diagnosis and continues thereafter. The methods for drawing insulin into a syringe, giving injections, and for insulin pen use are described in Chapter 8. Intensive insulin therapy (now standard treatment) consists of four or more injections of insulin per day or the use of an insulin pump, four or more blood sugar checks per day, and frequent contact with the healthcare team. Many people with type 1 diabetes eventually elect to use insulin pump treatment instead of multiple daily injections (Chapter 22). This often results in improvement in HbA1c levels, fewer severe low blood sugar episodes, and convenience in diabetes management.

Types of Insulin: The types of insulin are reviewed in Chapter 7. Initial therapy is usually with a basal insulin (Lantus, Levemir, Tresiba) taken once or twice daily. One of the three rapid-acting insulins, Humalog, NovoLog, or Apidra, is taken 15 to 20 minutes prior to meals or snacks and used to correct for high blood sugar levels.

Insulin for Meals: The pre-meal dose may initially be provided by the diabetes doctor using a "thinking" scale. This involves considering factors such as the blood sugar level, recent or planned exercise, and the type and amount of food to be eaten. Later, most people learn to base meal insulin dosages on carbohydrate counting (Chapter 4).

Correction Dose: The rapid-acting, short-lasting insulin is also used to correct high blood sugar levels (Chapter 11). The most common correction factor is one unit of insulin per 50 mg/dL (2.8 mmol/L) of sugar, initially correcting to a target sugar level of 150 mg/dL (8.3 mmol/L). Thus, with a blood sugar level of 300 mg/dL (16.7 mmol/L), a correction dose of three units of insulin would be taken to reach the desired blood sugar value. After the person is more experienced in diabetes management, lower target levels, particularly during the day, are often recommended. Additional doses can be given every one to two hours if needed.

NUTRITION

Chapter 3 outlines basic nutrition, which is important for everyone. Chapter 4 emphasizes eating nutritiously and introduces food plans (Constant Carbohydrate and Carb Counting). The appetite is often ferocious in the week or two after diagnosis, as the body weight is regained. Body weight then levels off and maintaining a normal weight and managing carbohydrate intake are major goals. **Portion size** is important in preventing excess weight gain. Avoidance of sugared soda and other junk foods high in carbohydrates is advised in the quest to normalize blood sugar levels.

The Constant Carbohydrate food plan is usually initiated at first (Chapter 4). With the Constant Carbohydrate Food Plan, about the same amount of carbs are eaten each day for a given meal. The insulin dose for food is then relatively consistent from day to day. Some variation in insulin dose from using a "thinking scale" can still occur (see Insulin for Meals on previous page). When ready, the person learns Carbohydrate (Carb) Counting. This involves counting the grams of carbs in foods to be eaten and matching the grams of carbs with rapid-acting insulin (Chapter 4).

Often, the dietitian requests a 3-day food record (Chapter 3) before selecting the insulin-to-carb (I/C) ratio. The initial I/C ratio is provided by the dietitian and physician. The most common I/C ratio is one unit of insulin per 15 grams of carbohydrate. This is then gradually adjusted based on the blood sugar levels after meals. It is recommended that all post-meal blood sugar values remain below 180 mg/dL (10 mmol/L).

BLOOD SUGAR (GLUCOSE) CHECKING

In contrast to people with type 2 diabetes, people with type 1 diabetes are expected to do four or more blood sugar checks per day starting on the day of diagnosis and thereafter. The number of blood sugar checks done per day clearly relates to optimal glycemic (blood sugar) control. The method for checking blood sugar levels is outlined in Chapter 9. The times for blood sugar checks are commonly in the morning upon awakening, before meals, sometimes one or two hours after meals, and always at bedtime. It is also important to check the level with any low blood sugar "reactions" (see Chapter 10). You should know the target blood sugar level to aim for when fasting in the morning (often 70-130 mg/dL or 3.9-7.27 mmol/L), and throughout the rest of the day (often 70-140 mg/dL or 3.9-7.8 mmol/L).

As noted above, all post-meal values should be below 180 mg/dL (10 mmol/L). Goals for blood sugar values should be discussed with your diabetes care-provider. Some adults with type 1 diabetes now use a continuous glucose monitor (CGM), which gives trends for changes in blood sugar levels as well as the current value (Chapter 23).

EXERCISE

Exercise is discussed in Chapter 5, and is important for all people. It helps in maintaining a healthy weight, improving one's mood, and in preventing cardiovascular problems. It also increases sensitivity to insulin, often resulting in lower insulin dosages and better sugar control. People with type 1 diabetes should always have a source of sugar with them when they exercise. Wearing a bracelet or other identification with the word "Diabetes" on it is also important in case of a low blood sugar, requiring help.

ACUTE COMPLICATIONS

Low Blood Sugar (hypoglycemia): Low blood sugar is discussed in detail in Chapter 10. People with type 1 diabetes who are receiving insulin are always at risk for low blood sugars. They must carry a source of sugar with them at all times. They should also have a glucagon emergency kit available in the home and workplace in case of a severe low blood sugar (Chapter 10). Family and associates need to be trained in how to use it. The use of CGM, with alarms for low glucose values, or for impending low values, can be very helpful in preventing hypoglycemia (Chapter 23).

Ketone Formation/Diabetic Ketoacidosis (DKA): Measurement of ketones and DKA is discussed in Chapter 12. Many people have ketones when initially diagnosed. It is then necessary to check the ketone level at regular intervals as advised by the diabetes care-provider.

Later, if insulin is missed (or a pump insulin infusion catheter is blocked/ not working), ketones will begin to climb after three hours. Every person with type 1 diabetes must have a method available (blood or urine) to check ketones, even during out of town trips. It is important to check ketones during any illness (even vomiting once). Ketone levels must always be checked if the morning fasting blood sugar is above 250 mg/dL (13.9 mmol/L) or anytime the blood sugar level is over 300 mg/dL (16.7 mmol/L). It is necessary when ketones are elevated to provide prompt administration of rapid-acting insulin by syringe, to drink extra fluids and to call the diabetes healthcare-provider if needed. It is much safer to prevent DKA than to have to treat it.

Treatment of Illness And Surgery: Treatment of illness (and surgery) is similar in people with type 1 or type 2 diabetes and is discussed in Chapter 13.

Frequent blood sugar and ketone checking is very important. Adequate fluid intake is a priority. A card with phone numbers of diabetes care-providers should be readily available.

PREVENTING CHRONIC COMPLICATIONS

Diabetes complications are discussed in Chapters 16 and 17 and are the same for type 1 or type 2 diabetes. The HbA1c level must be measured every three months (Chapters 2 and 19). If elevated (above 7.0 percent or 54 mmol/mol), steps must be taken with the help of the diabetes care team to get the value back down.

After type 1 diabetes has been present for two years, annual screening for kidney damage using the urine microalbumin level is important. Similarly, annual eye exams are advised. The likelihood of serious chronic complications is now very low if the HbA1c level is maintained below 7.0 percent (54 mmol/mol) (see Chapters 16 and 17).

The Diabetes Control and Complications Trial (DCCT) found several factors associated with optimal glycemic (blood sugar) control. These include:

- following some sort of meal plan
- not eating extra snacks
- not over-treating low blood sugars with too much food
- prompt treatment of high blood sugar levels when found
- adjusting insulin levels for meals
- consistency of bedtime snacks

PSYCH/SOCIAL

Many of the psych/social issues are similar for type 1 and type 2 diabetes. The need to learn to give insulin injections and do frequent blood sugar monitoring for people with type 1 diabetes initially adds extra time for education as well as increased stress. These factors are discussed in Chapter 14. Although getting diabetes can seem overwhelming at first, adaptation gradually improves. We recommend all newly diagnosed patients meet with the psych/social (psychologist or social worker) team members early on, and as needed thereafter.

SUMMARY

Much of the treatment of type 1 diabetes is similar to the treatment of type 2 diabetes. A major difference is the need to initiate intensive diabetes management at the time of diagnosis in ALL patients with type 1 diabetes. The frequency of insulin injections, blood sugar and ketone checking and the use of insulin pumps and/or CGMs are greater for people with type 1 diabetes. Having the best glycemic control possible is important for preventing diabetes complications for people with either type of diabetes.

FIGURE 1

Checking For Ketones

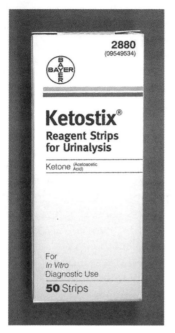

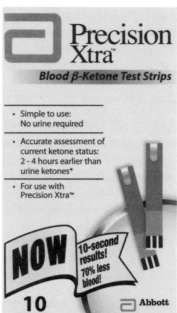

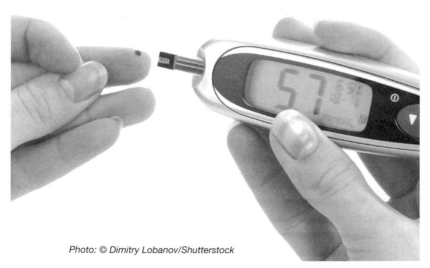

Photo: © Dimitry Lobanov/Shutterstock

Checking for urine or blood ketones with any illness or with high blood sugar levels is **VERY** important for people with type 1 diabetes (see Chaper 12).

AUTOIMMUNE CONDITIONS ASSOCIATED WITH TYPE 1 DIABETES

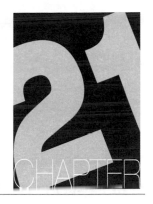

H. Peter Chase, MD, Loise A. Gilmer, MS, RD, CDE,
Satish K. Garg, MD

INTRODUCTION

O ther autoimmune (self-allergy) diseases are also associated with type 1 diabetes, but NOT type 2 diabetes. This is due to the inheritance of genes increasing the risk for autoimmunity that are also related to developing type 1 diabetes. Although there are many other diabetes autoimmune disorders, some of the more frequent conditions are thyroid disorders, adrenal disorders, celiac disease and skin problems.

THYROID DISORDERS

The thyroid gland, like the pancreas, is a hormone-producing organ. Thyroid hormones help to regulate metabolism (energy use). It is important for the diabetes care-provider to always check the size of the thyroid gland at each clinic visit. Some thyroid enlargement occurs in about half of people with type 1 diabetes, although only about one in 20 ever needs treatment. The reason for the enlargement is a similar "self-allergy" (autoimmune) type of reaction as occurs with type 1 diabetes. People who get diabetes often have an antibody in their blood against the insulin-producing cells in their pancreas (specifically, the islet cell antibodies, as discussed in Chapter 19). Likewise, people with diabetes who get thyroid problems usually have an antibody in their blood against the thyroid gland. This condition is called autoimmune thyroiditis (AIT). Relatives of people who have type 1 diabetes are also more apt to have AIT as a result of having the same high-risk autoimmunity genes.

The symptoms of low levels of thyroid hormone are variable. Some people feel tired all the time. Some people gain excessive weight.

If the gland is enlarged, specialized blood tests should be done, particularly a Thyroid Stimulating Hormone [TSH] level, as this is almost always the first test to become abnormal. If the TSH level is abnormal, it is recommended to repeat the level and to also evaluate other thyroid hormone levels.

If the thyroid tests show low thyroid function, a thyroid tablet can then be taken once daily. Thyroid problems are usually not serious unless unrecognized or untreated. The treatment is usually successful and involves taking pills (not shots).

Rarely, people with diabetes can have an overactive thyroid gland that produces excess thyroid hormone (hyperthyroidism). This can also be the result of autoimmune thyroiditis (AIT). Treatment by an endocrine doctor is then important.

ADRENAL DISORDERS

(Autoimmune Adrenal Insufficiency/ Addison's Disease)

The adrenal gland is a hormone-producing gland that sits on top of the kidneys. It produces several different hormones necessary to stay healthy, including cortisol, epinephrine and mineralocorticoids. Autoimmunity against the adrenal gland can also occur.

Adrenal autoimmunity is quite rare, occurring in about one in 500 people with type 1 diabetes, but it is important to diagnose and treat as it can result in death if untreated.

Cortisol, the hormone the body is unable to produce in Addison's Disease, is especially important during times of stress on the body, such as with an illness or injury. If Addison's disease develops, additional teaching will be required.

Some early signs for someone with adrenal disease may be:

- an increased frequency of severe low blood sugars

- episodes of feeling weak or faint with normal blood sugars, but sometimes low blood pressure

- two electrolytes in the blood, sodium (Na+) and potassium (K+), may be low and high, respectively

- later, darker skin coloring over the back of the hands, knuckles or elbows may occur

Initial screening may be for an antibody (21 hydroxylase antibody) against the adrenal gland. If positive, this should be followed by morning ACTH and cortisol blood levels (and an ACTH stimulation test, if needed). This can be discussed further with the doctor.

As with low thyroid hormone, the treatment of low adrenal hormone is with a tablet. Treatment includes training the person (or family) to increase the tablets during periods of stress (as with an infection or with surgery).

CELIAC DISEASE

Celiac disease (also known as gluten sensitivity, gluten-enteropathy or celiac sprue) is a genetically predisposed disorder in which the small intestine is damaged by an autoimmune reaction to gluten, a protein found in grains like wheat, rye and barley. The damage to the small intestine causes nutrients to be poorly absorbed.

The risk for celiac disease is carried on one of the genes (DR3) that is also related to being at high risk for type 1 diabetes.

Approximately one in 20 people with type 1 diabetes also has celiac disease. As other family members who do not have diabetes may also have the DR3 genetic type, they are also more likely to have celiac disease, even though they do not have diabetes.

It can be diagnosed using a blood antibody test (transglutaminase and/ or anti-endomysial antibodies). At present, an intestinal biopsy is often also done to confirm the diagnosis.

Symptoms may include:

- poor absorption of nutrients
- stomach pain
- gas
- diarrhea or constipation
- decreased height or weight gain in children
- iron deficiency anemia
- irritability
- dental enamel defects
- vitamin deficiency due to poor absorption
- osteoporosis

The symptoms, the abnormal blood tests, and the biopsy changes of the upper intestine may all return to normal within a few months after treatment is begun. However, this does not mean that the treatment can be stopped because the symptoms are likely to return.

TABLE 1

Grain, Seeds, Beans, Flours, and Cereals List for Celiac Disease

ALLOWED	Use with Caution	NOT ALLOWED
Amaranth	*Oats	Barley
Arrowroot		Bran
Buckwheat		Bulgur
Corn		Couscous
Flax		Durum
Hominy		Einkorn
Legume flours (bean, chickpea, garbanzo)		Emmer
		Farina
Millet		Farro
Montina™ (Indian rice grass)		Graham
		Kamut
Nut flours (almond, hazelnut, pecan)		Rye
Potato flour		Semolina
Potato starch		Spelt
Quinoa		Triticale
Rice		Wheat
Sorghum		Wheat germ
Soy and other beans		White flour
Tapioca		Whole wheat
Teff		

Oats cannot be guaranteed to be gluten free. Contamination can happen when oats are grown on the same field or processed in the same building as gluten containing grains.

Treatment:

- The only current treatment for celiac disease is strict adherence to a 100 percent gluten-free diet for life.

- Remove all wheat, rye, and barley products from the diet and any ingredient that contains these grains. Oats and oat products may also be removed from the diet initially.

- Many foods are naturally gluten-free and are allowed with the diet. These include rice, corn, potatoes, fruits, vegetables, meats and dairy products (see Table 1 for grains that are allowed).

The National Institutes of Health Consensus Development Conference suggested some elements needed in the management of Celiac disease.

C Consultation with a skilled dietitian

E Education about the disease

L Lifelong adherence to a gluten-free diet

I Identification and treatment of nutrition deficiencies

A Access to an advocacy group

C Continuous long term follow up by a multidisciplinary team

(NIH Consensus Statement on Celiac Disease. NIH Consens State Sci Statements. 2004 Jun 28-30 (1) 1-22.)

Other websites and possible helpful Celiac Associations are shown in the reference lists at the end of this chapter.

Skin Problems

- Yellow fatty deposits **(necrobiosis lipoidica)** can collect in the skin over the front of the lower legs. No one knows what causes these fat deposits, although they are most likely due to autoimmunity.

- A rare condition called **dermatitis herpetiformis** is also related to a sensitivity to the protein gluten (see celiac disease). It is characterized by blisters on the elbows, buttocks and knees. Like celiac disease, it responds to a gluten-free diet.

SUMMARY

Much is now known about the autoimmune problems associated with type 1 diabetes. Availability of gluten-free foods and information for people having celiac disease has expanded greatly in recent years. Autoimmunity is a relatively new area in medicine, and there is much on-going research.

REFERENCE LIST FOR CELIAC DISEASE
Celiac Associations & Advocacy Groups in the United States

Celiac Disease Awareness Campaign
National Digestive Diseases Information Clearinghouse
2 Information Way
Bethesda, MD 20892-3570
Phone: 800-891-5389
Internet: www.celiac.nih.gov

Celiac Disease Foundation
20350 Ventura Blvd., Suite #240
Woodland Hills, CA 91364
Phone: 818-716- 1513
Internet: www.celiac.org

American Celiac Disease Alliance
2504 Duxbury Place
Alexandria, VA 22308
Phone: 703-622-3331
Internet: www.americanceliac.org

Celiac Sprue Association/USA Inc.
P.O. Box 31700
Omaha, NE 68131-0700
Phone: 877-CSA-4CSA (877-272-4272)
Internet: www.csaceliacs.org

Gluten Intolerance Group of North America
31214 124th Avenue SE
Auburn, WA 98092
Phone: 253-833-6655
Internet: www.gluten.net

Academy of Nutrition and Dietetics
120 South Riverside Plaza, Suite 2000
Chicago, IL 60606
Phone: 800-877-1600
Internet: www.eatright.org

WEBSITES AND SUPPORT GROUPS:

www.celiac.com is an excellent site for safe/forbidden food additive lists, mainstream gluten free food products by brand name, gluten free recipes, discussion of controversial grains, etc. — and generally a good reference overall

www.glutenfreediet.ca; Shelley Case's (Expert Celiac RD) website with free patient education handouts, information on celiac disease and the gluten free diet

www.glutenfreedietitian.com Gluten-free nutrition updates, newsletters, and other resources for people with celiac disease

www.cdhnf.org Children's Digestive Health and Nutrition Foundation Can download: Gluten-Free Diet Guide for Families

www.glutenfreedrugs.com Lists gluten free drugs and vitamins and is maintained and run by clinical pharmacists

www.triumphdining.com Guide for eating out and grocery shopping

www.glutenfreemom.com website with good information for parents of kids with celiac disease

www.celiackids.com R.O.C.K: Raising Our Celiac Kids website support group

www.csaceliacs.info Celiac Sprue Association (CSA/USA): online support group for adults, parents, and kids (Cel-Kids Network)

BOOKS:

Gluten-Free Diet: A Comprehensive Resource Guide by Shelly Case, RD. www.glutenfreediet.ca

The Gluten-Free Gourmet Bakes Bread by Bette Hagman www.amazon.com or www.celiac.com

The Gluten-Free Gourmet Cooks Fast and Healthy by Bette Hagman www.amazon.com or www.celiac.com

Kids with Celiac Disease: A Family Guide to Raising Happy, Healthy, Gluten-Free Children by Danna Korn www.woodbinehouse.com

Incredible Edible Gluten-Free Food for Kids by Sheri L. Sanderson www.woodbinehouse.com

The Gluten Free Kid: A Celiac Disease Survival Guide by Melissa London www.woodbinehouse.com

Wheat-Free, Gluten-Free Cookbook for Kids and Busy Adults by
Connie Sarros www.amazon.com or www.celiac.com

**Pocket Dictionary: Acceptability of Foods and Food Ingredients
for the Gluten-Free Diet** Canadian Celiac Association www.celiac.ca

**Eating Gluten-Free with Emily: A Story for Children with Celiac
Disease** by Bonnie J. Kruszka www.amazon.com

MAGAZINES:

Gluten-Free Living: The Resource for People with Gluten
Intolerance. A newsletter available by contacting Gluten-Free Living,
P.O. Box 105, Hasting-on-Hudson, NY 10706.

Living Without: A Lifestyle Guide for People with Allergies and Food
Sensitivities_www.livingwithout.com

Delight Gluten-Free Magazine: Delightful Food, Delightfully Fun.
A bimonthly international food and lifestyle publication for people living
with food allergies and sensitivities.

INSULIN PUMPS

Laurel Messer, RN, MPH, CDE, H. Peter Chase, MD,
Satish K. Garg, MD

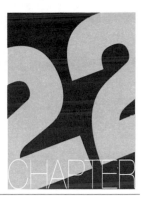

THE PUMP

An insulin pump is a pocket-sized device that continually administers insulin through a small tube that sits under the skin. It is commonly used in the treatment of type 1 diabetes and (rarely) in type 2 diabetes. Insulin pumps have become more popular in recent years. Advantages and disadvantages of pumps are discussed in Chapter 28 in the larger book, *Understanding Diabetes*, dealing primarily with type 1 diabetes. In addition, the book *Understanding Insulin Pumps and Continuous Glucose Monitors* is available (see "Ordering Materials" in the back of this book).

HOW IS INSULIN GIVEN BY THE PUMP?

It is important to note that an insulin pump can provide both basal insulin and bolus insulin (as discussed in previous chapters), but only uses a rapid-acting insulin (Humalog, NovoLog, or Apidra). Human Regular insulin is not used in pumps as it may block the infusion cannula. It is also not approved for pump use by the FDA.

The basal insulin is achieved by using a pre-set amount of rapid-acting insulin that drips slowly into the body every hour of the day. The pump automatically does this so the wearer does not have to think about manually giving basal insulin. This basal dose can be set to increase or decrease at different times of day as needed. This is one of the advantages of using an insulin pump over injection(s) of long-acting insulin.

A bolus dose is manually programmed by the insulin pump wearer. This is done whenever food is eaten or if a high blood sugar level is found. A bolus dose is calculated the same way with insulin pumps as it is with insulin injections, by using carbohydrate ratios and correction factors for high blood sugars. One advantage of the insulin pump over injections is that the ratios and correction factors are already programmed into the pump. The user enters a blood sugar level and the number of carbohydrates they plan to eat, and the insulin pump will automatically suggest the insulin dose. The person can then accept or alter the dose to be taken.

PARTS OF INSULIN PUMPS

All insulin pumps have the same basic components (see Table 1).

Insulin reservoir: All insulin pumps hold enough insulin to last for two to three days inside a replaceable insulin reservoir.

Control pad and display: The pump has a control pad with buttons for programming insulin delivery, either on the pump itself or on a remote device. It also has a display that shows current insulin doses, history, and many other settings.

Pump Body: Most insulin pumps combine their insulin reservoirs, control pads, and displays in a single unit called the "pump body." This is usually about the size of a cell phone or pager.

Tubing (except for the OmniPod®): Most insulin pumps are connected to the body with a thin plastic tube that comes in different lengths. The insulin is pumped through the tubing into the body. The OmniPod actually carries the insulin in a pod attached to the body and so does not need plastic tubing. The control unit is a wireless device, which is carried separately.

Cannula: All insulin pumps use a tiny plastic tube, called a cannula, inserted under the skin to deliver the insulin to the person. Each cannula is used for two to three days and is then replaced. There are different types of cannulas which come in different lengths and can be inserted at different angles.

Blood sugar meter: Many pumps can link (communicate) with a specific blood sugar meter. When that meter is used to check the blood sugar level, the result will be sent by radio-frequency to the insulin pump to help with insulin dosing. Some pumps have the blood sugar meter as part of the pump itself.

A list of the most common insulin pumps and features are found in Table 1.

TABLE 1

Features of Commonly Used Insulin Pumps*

Insulin Pump	Components	Keypad on pump or remote	Integrated or linked blood sugar meter	Other
Medtronic MiniMed Paradigm® REAL-Time Systems	Pump body, tubing, cannula	On pump only	Links to Bayer Contour® Next Link meter	Integrated with Medtronic Real-Time Continuous Glucose Monitor (CGM)
Animas OneTouch® Ping®	Pump body, tubing, cannula	On pump and also on One Touch Ping Meter Remote	Links to OneTouch Ping meter remote	Color screen
ACCU-CHEK® Spirit	Pump body, tubing, cannula	Simple keypad on pump, more features on ACCU-CHEK® Aviva Combo meter	Links to ACCU-CHEK Aviva Combo meter	Can bolus remotely from Aviva Combo Meter
Tandem® T-Slim	Pump body, tubing, cannula	On pump only	No	Color screen
OmniPod	"Pod" with insulin and cannula, separate PDM** with keypad and display	On separate PDM**	Integrated Freestyle® meter in PDM**	"Tubeless" system because insulin reservoir is inside pod attached to skin

*Websites for these five pump companies show pictures of the pumps and give more details:
- Medtronic (www.minimed.com)
- Animas (www.animascorp.com)
- ACCU-CHEK Spirit (www.accu-chekinsulinpumps.com)
- Tandem T-Slim (www.tandemdiabetes.com)
- OmniPod (www.myomnipod.com)

**PDM = "Personal Diabetes Manager"

WHAT IS INVOLVED WITH STARTING AN INSULIN PUMP?

Some facts about starting an insulin pump are outlined below.

- When you start an insulin pump you need to be proficient at carbohydrate counting and blood sugar checking. Both of these are essential to use the insulin pump safely.

- Before starting a pump, a diabetes care-provider will need to see your detailed records of blood sugar levels (at least four per day), food intake, and current insulin doses. This is needed to initially program the insulin pump to give the correct amount of insulin.

- Training for insulin pump use is usually done one-on-one with a Certified Pump Trainer and takes between two to six hours.

- The first one to four weeks of insulin pump use are the most difficult. As the system is learned, it becomes easier.

- Diabetes providers will want to see your blood sugar levels and pump information frequently during the first few weeks of pump use in order to fine-tune your pump settings.

- Bolus dosages for food are best taken 15-20 minutes before eating unless the blood sugar level is low or is trending low on a continuous glucose monitor.

- Table 1 gives an example of orders for insulin pump insulin dosages.

- Basal and bolus insulin doses are individualized for each person. The physician usually suggests initial basal rates. These can be fine-tuned as needed in order to provide the best blood sugar control.

- Close contact with the healthcare-providers is essential.

SOME ADVANTAGES OF INSULIN PUMPS

A few of the advantages of insulin pumps are outlined below:

- Insulin dosages can be adjusted for different periods of the day. This is true for settings of both basal and bolus doses.

- Insulin levels with exercise can be more safely managed (e.g., reducing or suspending basal insulin).

- Instead of giving frequent self-injections each day, the user has only to replace the pump cannula every two to three days.

- One pump (Medtronic), when used with a CGM, now has the property to automatically suspend insulin delivery at a set glucose level (Chapter 23).

- Several companies have recently developed patch pumps, including the Solo™ MicroPump by Roche Diabetes Care (for type 1 and type 2 diabetes), and the V-GO™ by Valeritas, Inc (for type 2 diabetes).

SOME CHALLENGES WITH INSULIN PUMPS

Pump challenges vary for different people, and may include the following:

- Starting insulin pump therapy initially requires extra training and a commitment from you and your family.

- As with giving injections, it is easy to forget to give bolus doses of insulin with high blood sugar levels or when eating.

- Because there is no long-lasting insulin working in your body, the pump is the only source of insulin. This puts pump users at higher risk for ketones and high blood sugar levels if the cannula (tube) comes out from under the skin or kinks. You must frequently monitor your blood sugar levels (and ketone levels if high) to avoid this.

SUMMARY

Insulin pumps are small devices that give both basal and bolus doses of insulin via a small tube under the skin. They can be programmed to administer different amounts of insulin for different times of the day. If you are ready to use an insulin pump, you need to be educated by a Certified Pump Trainer. Insulin pumps are most commonly used in type 1 diabetes but may also be used by people with type 2 diabetes.

TABLE 1

Insulin Doses

Name _____   Date*_____
                                  (*For insulin start)

STARTING BASAL RATE(S)

Start Time	Units per Hour	Start Time	Units per Hour
1._____	_____	7._____	_____
2._____	_____	8._____	_____
3._____	_____	9._____	_____
4._____	_____	10._____	_____
5._____	_____	11._____	_____
6._____	_____	12._____	_____

Total _____

CARB COUNTING
Starting Bolus Dosages

Time	Insulin/Carb Ratios	Time	Insulin/Carb Ratios
1._____	_____	3._____	_____
2._____	_____	4._____	_____

Insulin Sensitivity Ratio

Time	1 unit lowers BG by	Time	1 unit lowers BG by
1._____	_____mg/dl (mmol/L)	3._____	_____ mg/dl (mmol/L)
2._____	_____mg/dl (mmol/L)	4._____	_____ mg/dl (mmol/L)

TARGET BLOOD SUGAR LEVELS

Time	Target BG	Time	Target BG
1._____	_____	3._____	_____
2._____	_____	4._____	_____

Duration of Insulin Action: _____ Hours
If you have any questions, please contact your healthcare-provider:

MD: _____   Phone: _____

RN: _____   Phone: _____

Remember, you must call or fax blood sugar records in daily for the first 1-2 weeks after your pump start. Discuss this with your MD or RN at your Insulin Pump Start Visit.

CONTINUOUS GLUCOSE MONITORING (CGM)

Jaime Realoon, DC, H. Peter Chase, MD, Satish K. Garg, MD

O ne of the major advances in the treatment of diabetes in recent years has been in the development of the continuous glucose monitor (CGM). These devices give readings of subcutaneous (not blood) glucose levels every one to ten minutes. This compares with finger-stick blood sugar (glucose) readings which are usually done only four or five times each day. The subcutaneous CGM glucose values are approximately 10 minutes behind the blood sugar values, as the sugar must pass through the blood vessel wall into the subcutaneous space, and then the CGM system must determine the value. Considering the frequency of CGM readings, this delay has almost no clinical significance other than with symptomatic lows (see below).

The purpose of this chapter is to present a brief overview of CGM. An entire book on insulin pumps and CGM is available for people wanting more detailed information (*Understanding Insulin Pumps and Continuous Glucose Monitors* - see ordering materials in the back of this book). It is important to emphasize that, as with insulin pumps, the CGM technology is not for everyone.

- The person must want to use CGM and agree to use it consistently.

- Blood sugar levels must still be done at least twice daily to calibrate the CGM (see below). They must also be done anytime a low blood sugar is suspected and/or the CGM value is in question.

- CGM values will not always match the blood sugar values.

- It usually requires wearing the CGM at least six days per week to have an improved HbA1c value.

THE COMPONENTS OF A CONTINUOUS GLUCOSE MONITOR (CGM)

The CGMs currently available in the U.S. all have three basic parts.

Sensor: As with the insulin pump, a small plastic probe is inserted (with the push of a button) under the skin. The sensor reads subcutaneous (not blood) glucose levels for the next five to seven days (it is often possible to make them last even longer).

Transmitter: The transmitter attaches to the sensor and sends the glucose reading to the receiver.

Receiver or Monitor: The receiver is a mini-computer that collects, displays, and stores glucose readings. It receives information from the transmitter and converts the electrical signal to a glucose value in mg/dL or mmol/L. The MiniMed system (see below) has the receiver within the insulin pump (for pumpers). Sensor augmented pump therapy (CGM-pump) will likely become more common in the future, and include new ways to automate insulin delivery.

INITIATING CGM THERAPY

As with the initiation of insulin pump therapy, various clinics will have different protocols. The criteria for deciding who is ready to begin CGM therapy are similar to those for starting an insulin pump.

SOME ADVANTAGES OF USING CGM

Glucose levels: Knowing glucose levels every few minutes throughout the day, particularly after meals and during the night, can be a great help.

Trend graphs: The trend graphs show the direction glucose levels are going (in contrast to a single point in time for a blood sugar level). For people who use insulin, trend graphs can be VERY helpful for calculating the appropriate insulin dose.

Warning alarms: The alarms for high and low glucose levels, or for predicted high or low levels, can help to prevent episodes of DKA or hypoglycemia.

Lower HbA1c: If worn consistently (e.g., six days per week), HbA1c levels usually decrease.

Low Glucose Suspend (LGS)/Threshold Suspend (TS): One of the systems (Medtronic) now has a feature which allows the CGM to turn off insulin delivery from the pump if the CGM glucose values fall below a set level (often 60 mg/dL or 3.3 mmol/L). This is the first advancement in sensor-augmented pump therapy.

CHALLENGES FOR USING CGM

Adhesive issues: Adhesion problems for the sensor/transmitter are one of the two most frequent difficulties with CGM. For some people, this goes smoothly and is not a problem. For others, it is a major difficulty. These issues are discussed in detail in the *Understanding Insulin Pumps and Continuous Glucose Monitors* book (see order form in the back of book).

Calibration: In order to ensure the best accuracy possible, the CGM should be calibrated regularly to make sure that the sensor glucose readings are matching blood sugar values. Calibration involves doing a finger-stick blood sugar typically every 12 hours and entering the value into the receiver, preferably at a time when the blood sugar is not rapidly changing.

Alarms: Some people can be annoyed by the CGM alarms, or develop "alarm fatigue" and start ignoring them. Alarms can be set on "vibrate." If bothersome, discuss with the healthcare-providers.

Comfort: Inserting and wearing a sensor under the skin can cause skin irritation and discomfort. To make CGM use more comfortable, insertion devices are getting smaller and simpler to use.

Cost: Insurance coverage should be checked prior to ordering the CGM system. Coverage is gradually improving except for Medicare or Medicaid.

SENSOR PLACEMENT AND ADHESION

Placement: Each CGM company has suggestions for where to place their sensors. In general, they can be worn on the back of the arm, the abdomen, hips, or buttocks. The selected area must have enough skin/fat to be able to pinch up a little bit with two fingers.

Adhesive use: There are many different adhesive wipes, tapes, and bandages that can help sensors to stick to skin. It is quite common for a person to use an adhesive wipe to treat the skin under the sensor before placing the sensor on the skin, and then reinforce it with additional over-tape. Every person is different, and what works for one person may not work for others.

Most of the new sensors are approved for six-seven day use.

However, many patients extend the use of the sensor to 10-14 days by recalibration of the system ("off-label") use to save costs.

CGM DATA

There are two main types of data that can be obtained from CGM usage: Real-time and Retrospective. **Real-time data** refers to current data available while wearing the CGM (such as a "trend-graph" showing a series of glucose values). **Retrospective data** refers to past data that was collected and stored over time. Retrospective data can be accessed either by viewing trend graphs on the receiver display or by downloading the data to a computer. Each CGM system has its own cables and computer software for downloading retrospective data from the receiver. Both types of data are important and are explained in detail in the Pump and CGM book.

A COMPARISON OF THREE CGM SYSTEMS

Medtronic MiniMed REAL-Time Systems
(www.medtronicdiabetes.com)

Medtronic MiniMed has two similar systems available. Both systems use the Enlite sensor and MiniLink™ REAL-Time transmitter. The Enlite sensor is worn for six days before replacement. The sensor is inserted at 90 degrees using a spring-loaded automatic inserter that covers the needle during entry and removal. The **Guardian® REAL-Time system** consists of a typical CGM receiver, sensor, and transmitter. It can be worn by people who are not using an insulin pump.

The **Paradigm® REAL-Time System** consists of the same sensor and transmitter as the Guardian system, but it uses the MiniMed Paradigm Veo™ insulin pump as the CGM receiver. One advantage of the Paradigm REAL-Time system is the ability to use CGM and an insulin pump without having to carry two devices (insulin pump and CGM receiver).

The Paradigm Veo (called Minimed 530G® in the U.S.) is the first system to offer the LGS feature to prevent severe hypoglycemia. With the LGS feature, the CGM can be programmed to alert the user when the sensor glucose reaches a dangerously low level. If the user does not respond to the alarm, the Paradigm Veo will automatically suspend insulin delivery for two hours, or until the user cancels the suspension.

Dexcom™ G4 System
(www.dexcom.com)

The Dexcom G4 system has the smallest transmitter and the largest range of communication (20 feet). The sensor is worn for seven days before replacement. It is inserted using manual pressure rather than being spring loaded, so the user may control the speed of insertion. The sensors are placed at a 45 degree angle. The G4 receiver has a color-coded display to make it easy to quickly spot values above or below the user's selected target range. One disadvantage of the Dexcom system is that if the CGM user takes a medication containing acetaminophen (e.g., Tylenol®) while wearing the sensor, the CGM readings will be inaccurate (falsely high values) for a few hours.

Abbott FreeStyle Navigator®
(www.abbottdiabetescare.co.uk)

The Navigator sensor is worn for five days before replacement. The sensor is inserted at a 90 degree angle. The automatic inserter conceals the needle so that the user never sees it during entry or removal. A FreeStyle meter is built into the Navigator so that a second blood sugar meter does not need to be carried. The FreeStyle Navigator system was discontinued from the market in the U.S. in August 2011, but it is still available in Europe and many other parts of the world.

SUMMARY

The use of CGM is not for everyone. However, for many people who are ready and willing, the CGM can provide additional information, improve safety, and provide the potential for improved diabetes management.

TABLE 1

Features of Four CGM Systems

	Medtronic MiniMed Guardian REAL-Time	Medtronic MiniMed Paradigm REAL-Time Veo and Enlite sensor	Abbott FreeStyle Navigator	Dexcom G4
Parts of system	Sensor, transmitter, receiver	Sensor, transmitter, insulin pump	Sensor, transmitter, receiver	Sensor, transmitter, receiver
Communication between transmitter and monitor	6 feet	6 feet	10 feet	20 feet
Sensor life	3 days	6 days	5 days	7 days
How it obtains BG data	Bayer CONTOUR® LINK meter or manual entry	Bayer CONTOUR LINK meter or manual entry	Freestyle meter build into receiver	Manual entry
Initial warm-up calibration period	2 hours	2 hours	1 hour in 1.5 version	2 hours
Number of calibrations/day	2 per day	3 on first day, then 2 per day	5 in 5 days	2 per day
Frequency of real time readings	5 minutes	5 minutes	1 minute	5 minutes
Trend arrows	Yes	Yes	Yes	Yes
Hypo and hyper alarms	Yes	Yes	Yes	Yes
Predictive hypo/ hyper alarms	Yes	Yes	Yes	No
Rate-of-change alarms	Yes	Yes	No	Yes
Trend graphs	Yes	Yes	Yes	Yes
Downloading software	Yes	Yes	Yes	Yes
FDA approved: adults/children	Yes/Yes (pediatric version)	Pending	NA	Pending
Available in U.S.?	Yes	Pending	No	Yes

RESEARCH AND TYPE 1 DIABETES

INTRODUCTION

Banting and Best received the Nobel prize for their discovery of insulin in 1921. It was believed that a "cure" for diabetes had been found. Before the discovery of insulin, people with the more severe form (now called type 1 diabetes) lived only about one year after diagnosis. Insulin was not a "cure," but did save lives. Continued developments in the past three decades have resulted in great improvements in insulins, diabetes monitoring, diabetes control, lifestyle, and in the prevention of diabetes complications. Most people with type 1 diabetes can now live a normal life span if they have proper medical attention and strict adherence to care.

Four Common Research Questions

The four questions asked most often about research are listed below.

1. When will there be a cure?

2. Will there be a "bionic" pancreas?

3. Can diabetes be prevented?

4. Are there advances in preventing diabetic complications?

There has been wonderful progress in diabetes research over the last ten years. The next ten years will likely show even greater progress.

1. WHEN WILL THERE BE A CURE?

Islet Transplantation

In 2001, successful islet cell (the cells that make insulin) transplants were done in Edmonton, Alberta, Canada by Drs. A.M.J. Shapiro, E.A. Ryan, R.V. Rajotte and team.

All patients had "hard to manage" diabetes. Most were having severe insulin reactions (unconscious episodes or seizures) as a result of not recognizing lows ("hypoglycemic unawareness"). For this reason they were willing to take the three potent immunosuppressant medicines needed after receiving the transplant.

The most recent report on the "Edmonton Protocol" involved islet transplants in 325 adult recipients at many centers, sponsored by the National Institute of Diabetes and Digestive and Kidney Diseases (NIDDK) and the Juvenile Diabetes Research Foundation (JDRF). Three years after their first islet transplant (most had two transplants), 23 percent were insulin injection-free, and 29 percent, although back on insulin injections, were still producing some insulin. However, the results have been somewhat variable, and some centers have discontinued their programs due to patient complications. In addition, it has now been reported that the three initial immunosuppressant medicines used in the "Edmonton-Protocol" were causing kidney damage. Thus current research is focusing on the use of other anti-rejection medicines.

Dr. Bernhard Hering (University of MN) and his team have reported success for eight patients using just islets from one donor pancreas per patient. Their method of preparing the islets differs from the Canadian group. They are also using a new medication (an anti-CD3 antibody) to help prevent rejection. Five of their patients remained off insulin for more than one year. Some of the drawbacks to islet transplantation as a cure are summarized below.

- There are not enough human-donor islets.
- The medicines used to prevent rejection still cause side effects.
- The medicines must be taken for the person's lifetime.
- The medicines are costly.

Islet transplantation is currently used only in adults with diabetes that is hard to control. These people often have severe low blood sugars due to "hypoglycemic unawareness." With the advent of continuous glucose monitoring (CGM), it has been our experience that hypoglycemic unawareness can often be reversed. Some of the main goals for the future for islet transplantation involve:

- getting islets from an easier source (such as pig islets)
- continued evaluation of new medicines to prevent rejection
- investigating new methods to allow "tolerance" of the new islets so that potent immunosuppressant medicines do not have to be taken indefinitely
- protecting the transplanted islets from the person's immune system so diabetes does not reoccur

A group in New Zealand, under the direction of Dr. Robert Elliott, is using islets from one-week-old pigs for transplantation. The islets are covered with alginate (from seaweed) to prevent white blood cells (the immune system cells) from getting into the islets and destroying them. No immunosuppressant medicines are being used. Although this research is still in a preliminary stage, it does offer hope.

Whole Pancreas Transplantation

Type 1 diabetes can be cured by a whole pancreas transplant. It is important to remember that in people with type 1 diabetes, the immune system will also attack the transplanted tissue. The medications needed are the same as those given after any organ is transplanted (e.g., kidney, liver, heart). The medicines have improved but still have potential side effects. Some of these are:

- infections
- low white blood cell counts
- an increased risk for cancer

If a kidney transplant is needed due to kidney failure, so that the immunosuppressant medicines are needed anyway, a pancreas transplant may also be done. This may be done at the time of the kidney transplant or at a later time. Approximately 80 percent of the whole pancreas transplants are still functioning after one year.

Stem-Cell Transplants

Families frequently ask about hope from stem-cell transplants. Unfortunately, this is taking longer to develop than initially anticipated. It is not likely to result in a cure for diabetes in the near future.

In summary, the most important goal at this time is to keep in optimal blood sugar control. This will help prevent complications. Then, if a cure is feasible, the person will be able to benefit from it.

2. WILL THERE BE A "BIONIC" PANCREAS?

The "bionic" or "closed loop" pancreas refers to a combination of a continuous glucose monitor (CGM) sending glucose data to a mini-computer, which then instructs an insulin pump to give more or less insulin based on the glucose values. This is already partially available with sensor-augmented pumps. It will be some years, however, before complete "bionic" pancreas systems are approved for routine day-to-day use. This is due to many reasons, including difficulties with CGM accuracy at low glucose levels, the need to further develop computer algorithms (mathematical formulas) for insulin delivery, the need for a more rapid-acting insulin, and the Food and Drug Administration's (FDA) need to apprové such devices.

The Low Glucose Suspend (LGS), now referred to in the U.S. as Threshold Suspend (TS), a feature of the Medtronic Sensor Augmented Pump System, is already available and is described in Chapter 23 on CGM. This requires use of the Paradigm VEO (MiniMed 530G in the U.S.) insulin pump and the Enlite sensor with the Medtronic CGM. The LGS system represents a major advance in the development of the closed loop pancreas. The insulin pump is turned off for up to two hours if the CGM glucose value is below a set level (often 60 mg/dL or 3.3 mmol/L). This has been shown in four research reports to reduce time spent in hypoglycemia. It is an effective therapy to prevent severe hypoglycemic episodes.

Severe hypoglycemia is dangerous, and the ability to stop an insulin infusion from an insulin pump with a low CGM glucose level, or even better, with a pending low CGM glucose level, is very important. Approximately half of severe hypoglycemic events in adults occur during sleep. Thus, decreasing basal insulin or turning a pump off with actual or predicted hypoglycemia during the night is extremely valuable. The pump can be turned off for two hours without danger of ketone formation. Better warning alarms will also be valuable and are being developed.

3. CAN TYPE 1 DIABETES Be Prevented?

Prevention of Type 1 Diabetes

In many people it is now possible to predict that diabetes will occur. This is done by measuring the following antibodies in the blood:

- insulin autoantibody (IAA)
- GAD-antibody
- ICA512 antibody
- ZnT8 (Zinc transport antibody)
- fluorescent ICA antibody

Type 1 Diabetes/TrialNet (T1D/TrialNet)

The National Institutes of Health (NIH), with assistance from the Juvenile Diabetes Research Foundation (JDRF) and the American Diabetes Association (ADA), are supporting research aimed at preventing diabetes. The assumption is that if you can recognize who is at risk years before disease onset (which is now possible), then there must be some way to prevent the disease. A consortium of 12 centers in the U.S. and Canada and five centers in Europe and Australia are working together to identify people at high risk. Families having a first- or second-degree relative who started insulin treatment prior to age 40 can receive free screening for the above antibodies.

Some exciting initial data in relatives with high levels of insulin autoantibodies (IAA) suggests that diabetes can be delayed by six to nine years as a result of daily ingestion of oral insulin capsules. This research is now being repeated, and if similar results are obtained, could lead to many more studies. Families must agree to participate in this type of research if they wish to be able to prevent diabetes in future generations. The phone number to call to be screened is: 1-800-425-8361. More information is available on the website: www.diabetestrialnet.org.

The T1D/TrialNet consortium is also doing studies in people with recently-diagnosed diabetes to attempt to halt the destruction of the insulin-producing islet cells. It is now known that if a person continues to make some of their own insulin, the course of the diabetes will be easier and the eye and kidney complications (Chapter 16), severe low blood sugars (Chapter 10), and ketoacidosis (Chapter 12) will all be less likely. Several immunosuppressive medicines have already been found to have a temporary protective effect and these studies are continuing.

4. ARE THERE ADVANCES IN PREVENTING DIABETIC COMPLICATIONS?

The Good News!

The life span for people with type 1 diabetes continues to improve.

The main reasons for this improvement are due to the following:

- improvement in overall glucose control
- lessened risk of developing diabetic kidney disease
- kidney disease diagnosed at an earlier stage allowing reversal
- better management of high blood pressure
- treatment with lipid-lowering medicines, especially statins
- fewer people smoking cigarettes

The Bad News!

Some of the routine health evaluations and tests, such as kidney function tests, cholesterol levels and eye exams, are often forgotten, delayed or avoided. It is important for both the healthcare-provider and the patient to make sure that these tests are done regularly and any abnormalities treated quickly and appropriately.

Patient Responsibilities

If you have had diabetes for at least two years, **the two overnight urines should be collected every 12 months**. People often forget to bring in the overnight urine collection for the kidney-microalbumin screening to detect kidney damage (Chapter 16). It is important for the person with diabetes to remember to do this at regular intervals so that kidney damage can be caught early and treated appropriately. Directions for the collections can be found in Chapter 16.

As discussed previously, eye complications can also occur in people with diabetes. People with diabetes need to have regular eye exams by a diabetes-trained healthcare-provider.

Another important complication associated with type 1 or type 2 diabetes is cardiovascular disease (particularly heart attacks and stroke). This is discussed in Chapter 17. Optimal blood sugar control, not smoking, regular exercise and control of blood pressure and blood cholesterol are all important in the prevention of cardiovascular disease. Everyone must help take responsibility for their own health.

SUMMARY

The life span and quality of life for people with diabetes keeps getting better! This is due to better control of risk factors associated with complications, as well as to new medications and technologies. The delay, prevention, and safe cure of type 1 diabetes still remains a hope for the future.

TABLE 1

Type 1 Diabetes/TrialNet

People can call 1-800-425-8361 to find out the nearest place to go to obtain the free ICA screening test.

1. Screening Phase: Islet cell antibody (ICA) tests
The five antibodies that can be used in screening (see Chapter 3) are:
- GAD antibody
- ICA512
- IAA (insulin autoantibody)
- ZnT8 antibody
- Fluorescent ICA (if one or more of the antibodies listed above are present)

If one antibody is found, a second sample will need to be drawn to confirm the result. If the antibody is present in the second sample, then the person can enter the Monitoring Phase.

If more than one antibody is present, a second sample can be drawn for confirmation OR the person can go directly into the Monitoring Phase.

2. Monitoring Phase: The following tests are done:
- oral glucose tolerance test (OGTT) - to make sure diabetes isn't present
- islet cell antibody test (as described above)
- HLA (looking for the 0602 protective gene) at baseline visit only
- HbA1c

With all of the test results, the person can be provided with a risk level related to the development of diabetes (within the next five to ten years).

3. Oral Insulin Trial
Oral insulin was studied in the initial Diabetes Prevention Trial – Type 1 (DPT-1). Because a subgroup showed a favorable effect in delaying the onset of diabetes, a second study is now being done. The oral insulin trial is a double-blinded study in which the participants will receive either 7.5 mg of insulin or a placebo once daily and will not know which they are taking. The insulin taken by mouth does not have any low-blood sugar effect, as it is broken down into smaller particles by the stomach acid.

The participants in this trial have a 25-50 percent chance of developing diabetes in the next five years. In order to enter this study, the initial test results must show:
- a positive ICA test (x2)
- a positive IAA (insulin autoantibody) test (x2)
- normal insulin production on one IVGTT
- no protective genes (HLA-DQ 0602)
- a normal oral glucose tolerance test (OGTT)
- a mixed meal tolerance test (MMTT) is done shortly after entering the trial to determine the current level of insulin production

INDEX

PUBLICATIONS

Your purchase helps support Clinical Care and Research at the Barbara Davis Center for Diabetes. Thank you!

Item	Price	Qty	Total
Management of Diabetes in Adults 1ˢᵗ Edition	$15ᴬ		
Understanding Diabetes 12ᵗʰ Edition (The Pink Panther Book)	$20*		
A First Book for Understanding Diabetes 12ᵗʰ Edition	$12*		
Un Primer Libro Para Entender La Diabetes 11ᵗʰ Edition ("First Book" in Spanish)	$10*		
Understanding Insulin Pumps & Continuous Glucose Monitors 2ⁿᵈ Edition	$18*		
DIABETES: A History of a Center and a Patient	$15*		
Colorado residents add 7.75% sales tax	Tax		
SHIPPING AND HANDLING: $5.00 per book for orders of 1-9 books $2.00 per book for orders of 10+ books	S/H		
	Total		

Prices subject to change.

Name _____

Address _____

City/State/Zip _____

Phone _____ Cell _____

Email _____

❏ Please include me on the Children's Diabetes Foundation mailing list.

❏ Check enclosed payable to: Children's Diabetes Foundation
4380 South Syracuse Street, Suite 430
Denver, CO 80237

❏ VISA   ❏ Master Card   ❏ Discover   ❏ AmEx

Card # _____ Exp. Date _____

All orders must be paid in full before delivery.
Books are mailed USPS or Ground UPS. Allow one to three weeks for delivery.
Canadian and Foreign Purchasers: Please include sufficient funds to equal U.S. currency exchange rates.
For quantity order pricing and additional information call 303-863-1200
or visit www.ChildrensDiabetesFoundation.org.